Qigong

Suppleness and Strength Through Relaxation

(The Ultimate Beginner's Guide to Qi Gong Meditation and Healing)

Fredrick Walton

Published By **Phil Dawson**

Fredrick Walton

Qigong: Suppleness and Strength Through Relaxation (The Ultimate Beginner's Guide to Qi Gong Meditation and Healing)

ISBN   978-1-998038-03-9

No part of this guidebook shall be reproduced in any form without permission in writing from the publisher except in the case of brief quotations embodied in critical articles or reviews.

Legal & Disclaimer

The information contained in this book is not designed to replace or take the place of any form of medicine or professional medical advice. The information in this book has been provided for educational & entertainment purposes only.

The information contained in this book has been compiled from sources deemed reliable, and it is accurate to the best of the Author's knowledge; however, the Author cannot guarantee its accuracy and validity and cannot be held liable for any errors or omissions. Changes are periodically made to this book. You must consult your doctor or get professional medical advice before using any of the suggested remedies, techniques, or information in this book.

Table Of Contents

Chapter 1: Start on the Beginning

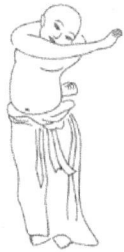

#1: Observe and take a look at who you would really like to be.

Take a have a have a observe the exquisite masters of Qi Gong, Tai Chi and unique martial arts. Those who're respected have had a extraordinary instructor, one they may test and emulate. Typically, pinnacle instructors of Qi Gong and Tai Chi martial arts are located and stated, each thru their college college students and thru the use of the people spherical them. So if there can be a person whom you recognize inside the world of Qi Gong, move and find out wherein they may be. If you could't bodily get to them, get pictures or video photos.

Study their movements and their behavioural styles.

In my sanatorium I in truth have a image of a Qi Gong hold close – an antique black and white taken inside the 1930s in San Francisco. It is some factor I even have a take a look at regularly. It facilitates me to preserve nicely shape in my Qi Gong workout. In particular, it permits me to recognition on my status postures.

One of my instructors, who is a long-term practitioner of Qi Gong and comes from America, recommended me that after he changed into meditating, his trainer used to sit down down a piece statue of Buddha coping with him. Whenever this instructor felt herself drifting or her very very own exercise waning, she might casually take a look at the Buddha, observe its shape, and function a study its form. This served to remind her to examine now not only the man or woman, but the individual's shape and behaviour, which can provide insight

2

into what makes that person a success every in working towards and coaching Qi Gong.

We are regularly blinded to our personal paintings and teachings. It's suitable to have a gentle reminder. So, are seeking out a teacher who is renowned and has a wide reputation. If you experience you have got determined that character, then sit down down and feature a examine. Observe how they educate, how they relate to their college students, examine their form, have a take a look at their posture, and pay attention to their desire of language. This is honestly the primary tip to get in advance. Treat this as a version by means of which you may formulate your own exercising.

#2: Practice at the least 20 minutes a day.

If you're going to be a Qi Gong instructor, you want to be ordinary. I apprehend for a fact that inside the years that I certainly have studied and finished guides at one-of-a-kind faculties, this purpose has been the hardest for me to gather. It took me four years to apprehend that everyday exercising, although it's nice twenty mins a day, is manner greater beneficial than schooling a few times a week for an hour.

The primary concept in the lower back of this is that normal practice hones your Qi glide, easy as that. We comprehend that surely each person who is on the top in their pastime in any issue is schooling always. This maintains the tough wiring of the brain in location, stops it from demise out and guarantees that electricity doesn't reduce. So, make it your mantra that twenty mins every day is higher than an hour as quickly as each week, and take into account the Chinese pronouncing: 'One day with out workout, you observe it. Two days without workout, your teacher notices it. Three days without workout, your university students be aware it.' Be consistent in your art work and it will shine through.

#3: Don't be worried to steal thoughts from your instructor.

Now that doesn't advocate stealing their system and making it your very own. What you could do, but, is borrow any thoughts, actions, stances, and meditations that resonate properly with you. Any proper Qi Gong instructor or practitioner can also have had at least one or right instructors of their existence. Some teachers can also have greater of a yang technique and some extra of a yin approach to their coaching. You can draw from each elements.

For instance, I definitely have 3 Qi Gong instructors within the meantime. One of them I may liken to a tiger. He's lithe, muscular, and robust, however is really pretty smooth in his movements. There is nearly a mild stalking to his approach. He seems to creep up on you for the duration of the artwork until the prevent of an afternoon-long workout, while he pounces with a completely closing lesson that genuinely hammers the studying home and consolidates the artwork.

I simply have every other instructor who's extra like a monkey. He may be very playful and earthy and likes you to find out the paintings. He is not a lot arms on, however is greater language-primarily based completely and really a good buy focuses on your shape, frame language, posture, and hand gestures inside the path of the paintings. So it's a very exceptional fashion, but further surprising. In a manner, it allows you to self-find out the art work because of the truth irrespective of what number of books or scriptures or films on Qi Gong that you see, you don't take a look at it till you revel in it. Take from the schooling and teachers who virtually resonate with you. Borrow those thoughts, 'scouse borrow' them and incorporate them into your non-public artwork. Because in case your very private instructor is brilliant, she or he is brilliant for a purpose and you can eliminate subjects that you could discover will resonate well together together with your college college students. They will be conscious this resonance, surely. Bear in mind additionally that imitation is the extremely good form of flattery, so in a manner you're honestly doing a company to the paintings. You're allowing your teacher's artwork to preserve in some shape of ancestral lineage.

#4: Keep a diary of all your thoughts, insights and observations.

Do this no longer simplest inside the course of your very very very own exercise, but additionally at the same time as you are schooling college university college students. As any pinnacle athlete will inform you, at the same time as they're education or building up for a competition they keep a diary, then they're able to cognizance on what the highs and lows are as well as the versions a number of the 2.

For instance, did the immoderate or low element rise up at the identical time as you have got were given been education/schooling, or have been outside forces appearing on you? Where became your electricity within the path of your exercising? Had you overlooked an afternoon or had you been unwell? All these observations are essential due to the reality they will be the key to unlocking your true capability as a trainer and therefore helping you to realise the identical kind of highs and lows for your university college students. Keeping a diary moreover permits you to preserve a ancient account of the way you've superior as a teacher, so you can appearance decrease lower back in 3 or four years and spot in that you have been once more then and evaluate it to in which you're now. Sometimes from the past there can be training you may deliver forward into the destiny and on occasion mind/thoughts you had on the time weren't appropriate if you want to use, but now, 4 or five years later, they may be perfect as a way to comprise into your non-public exercising and education. There are extra treasured schooling in a diary of your very very very own existence than many one-of-a-kind training you may look at. Note the changes that arise, the schooling you've observed out, and the thoughts which have come into play. Perhaps you haven't had a hazard to deliver them to fruition. One instructor used to mention to me, 'Ideas are like wet fish; in case you don't keep directly to them they'll slip thru your arms.' Writing down your studies is a manner to keep onto your training, song your evolution, and revisit thoughts.

#five: Be organized to make errors.

It's k to make mistakes. It's right enough to be imperfect. It's suitable sufficient for you to be ok with that. However, that's not to mention you need to be lazy approximately it. Don't be afraid to inform your college students when you do make a mistake. Your university students will recognize that you are simplest human, even if you are the very pleasant Qi Gong draw near of your device.

Mistakes are part of being human. Another trainer used to say to me, 'Mistakes are gadgets given to you to study.' Don't beat yourself up approximately the minor stuff. It's an opportunity so one can see wherein you're at in the gift second, so that it will take stock and in all likelihood refine the art work which you are doing. It additionally shows your university college college students that you're going through your very very personal manner. They will understand you for that, and on your honesty. If you train them a selected manoeuvre, stance, or series of moves, and you are making a mistake midway via, don't try to overcorrect it. You are higher off apologising and moving in advance, because of the fact that hassle or that mistake has been dealt with, correctly and efficiently. There are not any hidden agendas and it maintains the strength flowing whilst you are education. I am a robust believer no longer in allowing mistakes to appear, however in accepting that they every so often will, and when they do, I welcome them, display them, and allow them to skip.

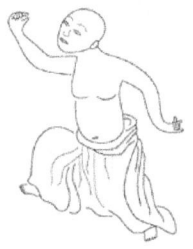

#6: Teach in easy settings.

Your Qi Gong isn't going to be any greater due to the reality you're doing it in a elaborate spa inn or a seashore excursion motel in choice to a pleasant, simple log cabin inside the woods. Some of my favored Qi Gong periods were executed inside the close by park with buddies and co-people. In reality, an entire lot of the places wherein I located out Qi Gong have been unpretentious rooms, regularly designed for teaching normal such things as flower arranging or origami.

Simple settings are more conducive to gaining knowledge of. If there's too much fluff, you'll discover that scholars can be distracted thru manner of the surroundings. This is right of many particular structures. Over the years I've educated in severa types of martial arts in addition to Qi Gong and some of the extremely good commands I've had were in simple brick homes in China with smooth matting on the floor. The domestic home windows didn't even have glass in them. There were really pretty simple scriptures and scrolls at the wall. So, schooling in a humble setting gets rid of the clutter out of your mind and from your college university college students' minds and allows space for the Qi Gong teachings to arise. Let that be a lesson for your university college students moreover;

permit them to create region for themselves in a clean placing.

In the beginning some college college students, especially individuals who are doing Qi Gong extra as a hobby instead of a way of existence, typically generally tend to locate themselves doing Qi Gong inside the front of the TV, or while the radio is on. Those who are a touch more crucial about it have a tendency to awareness on a nicer placing, such as the decrease again garden or the nearby park, or a room within the residence that they set aside specifically for exercising. A clean putting is better. It approach an lousy lot plenty much less distraction and further reputation. Often you may locate in records some of the first-class gyms and martial arts training halls and dojos were very humble locations truely. Not much like the contemporary-day day gyms which can be very cerebral, very focused on loud music and mirrors and machines. Keep it easy. It's regularly the much less tough putting that creates the less tough Qi Gong and in my experience, the greater clean the Qi Gong, the extra hard it is and the greater the reward.

#7: Don't be concerned to mix styles at the same time as you're schooling.

Mix your hard and gentle techniques collectively. Don't be troubled of mixing smooth Nei Gong and difficult Qi Gong patterns collectively due to the truth from time to time you could discover there can be a extra gain for the scholar in the event that they see every aspects of the artwork. Sometimes this mixture of difficult and mild patterns not quality relates to the shape of Nei Gong or Qi Gong that you are teaching, however moreover in your method to the teaching. Don't be fearful to be a touch bit militaristic. Be strict and strong – push your university students alongside and train them – but moreover don't be anxious to step again within the same splendor and turn out to be easy, slight, and nurturing. You'll be

14

amazed which college college college students broaden higher with a stronger method and which amplify better with a softer, more nurturing method. It's accurate for the scholars to experience each factors of that coaching, it permits them to improvement and to shape their very very personal critiques approximately Qi Gong, and possibly determine how they would really like to educate it themselves.

The difficult and smooth forms of education have been taught to me via various humans so I've had teachers with a extra hard technique, a stricter extra disciplinary approach, after which other teachers who had been softer and similarly nurturing. So I virtually have skilled each the difficult and clean forms of gaining knowledge of and I see benefits in each. Teaching tough and smooth collectively allows you to get right of access to specific quantities of someone's psyche. It makes you a greater rounded instructor and it moreover suggests your university college students that at the same time as on occasion you'll be a soft touch, you may be a difficult undertaking grasp when you need to be. You earn a more feel of appreciate for that; they recognize which you are immoderate approximately the paintings.

#eight: Teach the greater hard patterns with precision.

If you're coaching the harder fashion of Qi Gong for strengthening the body (together with the viscera, bones, and tissues), there needs to be a greater amount of precision on your schooling, bodily and energetically. You want to be laser-like to your method, be thorough, and be really unique approximately the exact movements that need to take region and the right series on your college students to perform them in, so as for them to maximise the advantages in that form of exercise. The very last thing you need is on your college university college students to be doubtful about the manner to do your precise style of Qi Gong. Lack of precision can also cause possible accidents or infection. If you may train tough patterns, teach with precision, train as if you are coaching them the way to perform surgery.

#nine: Teach the softer patterns with gentleness.

If you are focusing on the gentle abilities, the ones greater like Nei Gong or an internal exercising wherein you are softening the breath and softening the moves, allow the movements to move deeper, past the tissue, into the Qi of the frame, into the organs. Teach that with a smooth technique.

Each individual has a exceptional energetic signature, a great psyche, a specific manner of life, a splendid upbringing, probable even a awesome diet and a superb cultural impact. So in case you're going to move inner, if you are going to melt the artwork, permit space for self-exploration. Allow them to enjoy, explore and precise, each verbally and bodily, what it is they want to exercise consultation through their system. This method will assist them consolidate in their very personal thoughts what the artwork of Qi Gong and Nei Gong technique to them and the way it relates to them internally as a person. You're giving them area to transport inner. Don't underestimate the electricity of walking softly; it may have a greater a protracted way-attaining and profound effect than some of the more tough techniques to schooling.

#10: Prioritise tough abilities to come to be more potent.

If you need to grow to be a stronger teacher and a stronger practitioner of Qi Gong, prioritise hard talents as your foundation. You need a sturdy shape if you want to emerge as stronger internally. If you want to come to be higher at something – whether or not or no longer or now not it is Qi Gong, sports, remedy, or your every day existence as someone – make the more hard Qi Gong competencies, which incorporates the status postures and the outside manifestation of the work, your basis. Hard skills red meat up your bones, your tissues and your alignment, so it could be the form of Qi Gong that works the tendons, the bones, the muscle agencies, the breath and the diaphragm. Have those as your basis so they may be a part of your each day exercise at some diploma. Don't turn out to be too reliant on the smooth competencies, because of the fact without proper shape and without right form, the Qi Gong acquired't drift efficiently or to its fullest ability and you then are possibly missing out on a deeper layer of transformation within the artwork that you carry out as a instructor. No one desires to go to a trainer who seems ill or out of shape. And recall me, inside the Qi Gong international there are some of teachers who're out of form.

#11: There are not any prodigies in Qi Gong.

There are simply humans who've mounted a whole lot of strive and some of difficult paintings. I'm constantly a piece bit sceptical of all of us who calls themselves a hold near, because of the truth who absolutely has the right to name themselves the keep close of a few thing? We're continuously mastering at the same time as we're proper right here on the planet. Any time I've met a person who has been referred to as a baby prodigy, of Qi Gong, martial arts or of every other capacity, which consist of piano gambling, for example, they'll be normally formed by using an out of doors detail, typified through their surroundings. They're now not clearly born prodigies. They start at a totally more younger age and are commonly uncovered to a miles extra disciplined surroundings of normal and prolonged exercise. Don't beat yourself up about not achieving ranges as rapid as you want. Anyone you agree with you studied is a prodigy is someone who had an environmental benefit.

#12: How to choose your very personal teach.

Anyone who's proper at something — whether or not or no longer it is martial arts or Qi Gong or clay-pigeon taking pix — has had a teach. However, you need to pick out the right one for you. If you'll be an remarkable teacher of Qi Gong and be reputable, respectable, and loved in your artwork, at the back of you desires to be a person who is liable for your workout and skills on the same time as preserving you focused and down to earth. This goes for being a practitioner too, no longer in reality instructors.

Look at a number of the arena's pinnacle golfers, snooker gamers, or footballers — all of them have a key issue: an first rate train.

A teach desires to mission you, confront your willing regions, and preserve you liable for your schooling. I excursion every few months to fulfill with my teachers to make sure I am being held chargeable for everyday workout; they can see it in me, they may take a look at me like a book, they understand if I've been a chunk off in my schooling or if I've had down time or if I've made one too many excuses. But it's brilliant, as it receives me decrease returned on the right tune – I recognize I simply have someone searching out for me.

These expectancies can enlighten your university university college students, developing and recycling excellence on the equal time as passing for your coaching ethos.

Chapter 2: Find the Edge

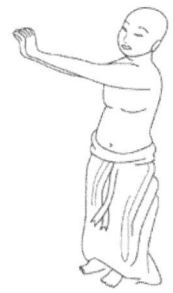

#13: Find the threshold.

When teaching Qi Gong, Tai Chi, inner arts, or anything energy art work you are concerned in, you've got to find out the brink interior your training. The side is the potential to take your university students to that uncomfortable spot wherein they benefit notion into wherein they want to be in their education. If they need to make a distinction to their very own health, nicely-being and exercise, finding the threshold will assist to get them there.

This is completed through way of way of slowly constructing up the momentum and strain inside the paintings you're demonstrating, then – over a time period interior that beauty, or internal a few commands – taking your university university college students a chunk in the direction of the issue of soreness, the place in which they simply enjoy what it's like. For instance, if we select out to do a standing posture, understanding that on average maximum college university students can also best be reputation for a period of ten or fifteen mins a day, take them to the aspect in which they may be virtually protective on for the previous few minutes. They can do it, they apprehend they are capable of do it, however they've in no manner earlier than been taken to that vicinity wherein they enjoy they've been recognition for forty mins. It's an success, it's an accomplishment. It's like if you have been education in popular sports activities sports like soccer or athletics and all at once realised that truely to play those brief even as extra isn't going to motive you any more problem, or do any greater harm to your body, or have an impact on your strength tiers, however instead will take you to a place in that you recognize that you can normally push yourself that little bit similarly.

In a classroom environment, you're had been given a first rate advantage in taking your university college students to that vicinity. You want to avoid frustration, anger or resentment. Students need to revel in they've been demonstrated with utmost readability the level they need to be performing at to get the maximum advantage. On occasion, additionally they need to discover the threshold in their very very own exercising. The high-quality way of helping them to accumulate this is with the useful aid of guiding them to that location to start with. Rest confident, they will be watching you and seeing in that you're at. You furthermore want to make certain that in case you will take your university university college students to the threshold, which you keep beforehand of them in your personal degree of Qi fitness.

#14: No clock searching.

No clock searching while you're training. It is quite not unusual for instructors to set up a timer, and that's first-rate, I haven't any issues with that, but to your very own workout attempt to keep away from clock searching. It creates an environment in which the pupil is not present collectively with your coaching, they may be generally dashing in advance and wishing the time away. That character will coast through or carry out the obligations or positions with little hobby.

If there's a elimination of the emphasis at the clock, they may apprehend that with a excellent, robust, present exercise and full engagement with the art work, the time passes effortlessly. Occasionally twenty mins will appear to be high-quality 5. At one of a kind times, it's the possibility manner spherical. This shows wherein the character is in their private fitness.

Another reason for removing the clock is that it can split the elegance waft. Ultimately this disrupts the Qi and might destroy the relationship you have got got were given along with your students on an strength diploma. The clock is a beneficial device within the starting for some college college students because of the reality they may gauge the length of their exercise with the aid of it. However, it doesn't gauge the intensity of their exercising. The rate you are trying to impart to them about the clock is that a few humans can stand for an hour, however it's the top notch of the reputation that's critical. It's an prolonged way higher to face for twenty minutes in a deep, easy, related Wu Ji posture. Standing for an hour in a half of-hearted try at a stance confers far masses less benefit than from a complete connection.

#15: Chunking it down.

Break down your training. This is so critical, I emphasise it over and over while education. You can also moreover have a form you want to impart on your college students. It can be a form of 100 actions, a hundred and 80 moves, thirty actions or seven moves. It's a long way extra for you as a instructor to take sections of this shape and spoil it down into person movements. These person movements can be taught as a form of Qi Gong of their very personal proper. It builds up recognition, understanding, and familiarity with the tool. It additionally makes the challenge lots less overwhelming for you as a teacher if you have a number of paintings to hold to the desk. If you're coaching at retreat and there's a sure level of hard work that desires to be imparted, it's lots higher in case you take the extra complicated moves of that Qi Gong art work and damage it down into additives. So, for example, in the university in which I teach and train, we workout the dragon form. The dragon has quite some of motion and sequences, a number of which can be easy and familiar to my college students on the identical time as others are more complicated.

I take the extra complex actions and repeat them over a period of hours during the training. Ultimately, university college students end up very acquainted with the ones styles of actions. To teach extra complicated actions I take each segment/subsection of that motion and destroy it down even further. Then we coaching, as an instance, the arm moves in the dragon, then the arm and foot moves, integrating the centre motion with the arm, toes and body movement. Suddenly a few issue which seems hard to educate may be put together simply and grow to be far extra apparent to the scholar. Instead of looking to teach one complex motion in a repetitive style until they nail it, (that could every now and then take months for them to gather) college college students can see themselves progressing extra rapidly.

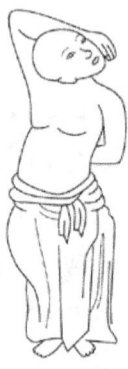

#sixteen: Building perfection.

This follows on properly from 'Chunking it down'. Build perfection into now not only your teachings, however additionally the varieties of movements you're training your college college students. You can exceptional construct perfection collectively with your university students one glide at a time. There's no factor in seeking to educate seven or 8 actions proper now, due to the fact the mind isn't going as a way to technique it if it's a cutting-edge-day motion. Students want to research one motion or one segment of one movement at a time, grow to be familiar with that movement/posture and be capable of repeat it without a cause sight. So you're respiration a few familiarity into not nice the bodily, however additionally the metaphysical, with the primary involved tool. It is important for university youngsters to recognize the concept of perfection and to want to nice their paintings. It does require, as with a few aspect associated with schooling and coaching, ordinary art work of a repetitive nature.

When you spoil every motion down, the pupil will begin to apprehend the subtext and to understand the subtlety and complexity inner that movement. There's a saying inside Qi Gong and is the cause that during case you've got got a test the microcosmic, you'll have a more knowledge of the macrocosm, and vice versa, so reading the macrocosm gives you an facts of the inner dynamics of the microcosm. It's a profound philosophy which desires to be covered into the paintings to allow the scholars to benefit a level of perfection. It is also an top notch way of training ethically in that you are setting the identical vintage to your students from the start.

#17: Embrace pain.

Many people come to Qi Gong with a completely idealistic view of it. They bear in mind it as a whimsical Chinese philosophical/medicinal difficulty which offers all of the benefits of Chinese remedy without any of the discomforts that go with special styles of workout. Now, to a positive quantity this is proper. Certain stages of strain/trauma which can be because of excessive pace, immoderate effect wearing events were removed. But you need to make your college university college students conscious that Qi Gong does require a sort of fitness and interior that shape of health there will be a diploma of ache as they get used to the physical sports.

Typically, I allow my college college college students to experience pain, to consist of it. I allow them to apprehend that that is the body letting bypass. There is usually a large amount of ordinary and hereditary tension in the body form. Qi Gong lets in a connection which permits the student to awareness on areas that could want more artwork. Part of that is to enjoy discomfort. It has to revel in like paintings, it has to revel in like a few quantity of attempt is wanted in advance than the payoff. I count on possibly the maximum tough and uncomfortable difficulty to comprehend is meditation, in all likelihood seated meditation, and especially seated mediation on a ground or mat, in an upright function, lotus style. This can display to be a actual undertaking for an entire lot of college college students, now not most effective mentally, but bodily too. It's very critical which you take them to that location and permit them to embody that degree of soreness. As their fitness improves, due to the reality the spine and joints open and their power begins offevolved offevolved to go with the go together with the float, they begin to revel in a bargain less ache.

#18: Be steady in your personal workout.

What does this mean? Well, it technique practising constantly and regularly, for a term, because the frame and thoughts like repetition. Being normal on your exercising brings constant Qi glide and builds robust shape. It strengthens your will and teaches you field. Being consistent approach that you are constantly related, you're constantly tuned in to the Qi, so that you have a reserve for even as you want it maximum.

#19: Practice on my own.

As a train and trainer, you need to encompass the philosophy of being cushty with your self and the art work, with none distraction, remarks, or out of doors forces which may also moreover intervene alongside aspect your mindfulness.

Practicing on my own regularly builds self-self assurance and self-popularity without outside effect. Typically, some college students might be used to training in organization settings, with possibly some exercise at domestic. As a trainer you need to encompass the philosophy of the vintage masters, it's miles 'don't be afraid to take off, get a while away, exercise by myself'. The more you exercise this philosophy, the extra you can resonate together together with your non-public power. Use yourself-focus. Manipulate your energy without every person drawing on you. It will come up with a sense of tranquillity, of peace, of connection, and will let you harm any lively connections with outdoor dynamics that may be taking location within the company you are education, or internal your very own exercising. Practicing on my own lets in time for internal recognition, and to mirror at the paintings you've been doing at the side of your university college students.

#20: Don't be afraid to use photographs.

All university college students observe otherwise — some are seen, others are extra kinaesthetic, some auditory. Imagery is a form of talking with the subconscious thoughts. I normally inform my college college students that a number of the extraordinary Qi Gong teachers and some of the incredible Qi Gong practitioners are humans with cool animated film minds who can conjure up photos. Using pix allows you to glimpse the 'yi', that is your popularity. Visualise, as an example, which you're status in an earth posture. Imagine a large mountain in the lower back of you; have a have a examine that mountain, its form, its period, its energetic glide, its depth, its warmth, its coldness, its earthiness, its rockiness — all of those specific elements come into play.Visualisation lets in you to hyperlink into that part of the mind that is acquainted with that form of language greater with out difficulty. I do believe imagery internal schooling enables college college students to assemble into their art work a deeper know-how and connection; it focuses the mind on what they're doing. There can be instances at the same time as a number of the scholars received't have that shape of reference to what they will be doing. Then you may should keep in mind what it's far they're feeling, whether or not or not they're feeling a vibration, yi, bloodless, warm — what are the sensations they may be tapping into inside the paintings. Play at the aspect of the sensations they'll be feeling until they reconnect with the artwork. Reinforce and bolster that connection thru encouraging robust visualisation. Simply positioned, use photographs to help, now not handiest with your training/training but moreover together collectively together with your exercising.

#21: Pay hobby to mistakes.

If you're making a mistake, put your hand up. Don't be worried as a instructor to mention, 'Ah, I made a mistake there, I'll correct it.' You'll get far more understand for that. Your students will see that you're no longer invincible, you're human. They'll see that you are to your very very personal adventure and it will prevent a construct-up of resentment or confusion. Clarify your factor, understand your college students.

If you gift the work in a single way and you're making a mistake, and then you definately present it in a extraordinary manner with out remark, the pupil is left asking the question, 'Well, which way is it completed?' You ought to make certain that in case you've made a mistake, you're saying, 'OK, yeah, I did that incorrect. Let's honestly skip over that another time.' This has passed off to me in elegance and it has befell to me in China once I've been training with vintage masters who've been supplying the paintings.When a mistake is made a knowledgeable extra youthful scholar will say, 'Well, in reality, no draw close, it is going this way,' and stated the grasp can also reply, 'Oh, yes, certain, that's proper,' this is splendid. Other masters may moreover say, 'Oh, don't be so insolent, don't talk to me like that. This is the way we're doing it in recent times.' This is due to the reality they've built themselves as an awful lot as be a huge legend of their very own proper and they don't need to be visible to be incorrect. This may be quite a commonplace prevalence with some instructors, no longer best in Qi Gong but in different disciplines as nicely.

So, as a trainer be aware of your mistakes and be aware of your university students' mistakes. Don't permit them to interrupt out with mistakes, because of the truth mistakes end up recurring, then it will become very hard to be able to re-sample, to introduce the proper moves. This doesn't advocate being crucial, it really technique ensuring that you have taken word of the mistake, you've got were given highlighted it, and you're supplying answers or new methods of correcting the ones mistakes.

#22: Visualise yourself as a pupil.

This may be very beneficial to instructors and teachers of Qi Gong. Put yourself in a study room putting as a scholar and visualise yourself being taught. Imagine yourself taking on board the facts and absorbing it, energetically, bodily, through auditory or vibrational channels. See the power of the training going into your body. Don't be concerned to position your self into the scenario of a pupil and spend time reflecting on how you will research if you had been coaching your self. Make some notes on it because of the truth it could be a completely valuable device.

#23: Visualise yourself changing.

This frequently helps with university college students who require motion, exchange, recovery or development inside the artwork. Here's an example I regularly use once I do a standing mediation. It calls for my college college students to internalise through last their eyes and visualising their backbone as a column. I inform them that it doesn't need to be anatomically accurate or best, however surely to get a revel in visually or bodily of what their backbone looks as if, from the top all of the way all of the way all the way down to the tail bone.

They learn how to visualise the regions which can be slight, dark, murky, foggy, incredible, vivid, or some thing functions they'll personal. Then I ask them to do some sort of motion, some form of clearing Qi Gong, some centreline movement, and to connect with clearing, with changing, with reworking. I ask them to visualize themselves clearing out the gunk, dredging the impure strength from the body, then in the end returning to the meditation, going internal and looking what adjustments have took place.

Visualising change is a totally effective shape of recovery and learning. You will do nicely to consist of this into your very own teaching workout. This kind of art work isn't always without troubles imparted by using some of the Chinese masters I've knowledgeable with. Many of the more esoteric or visualisation mind are not constantly without troubles distributed to Westerners. There are some mind which want to receive to Westerners in a Western context. Visualising alternate, but, is a effective manner of bringing it into the students' focus.

#24: Practice in constrained areas.

Students can be able to experience the difference within the strength amongst an open room and a closed room. It creates depth with the studying, which is pretty transformative. It teaches the students the way to go along with the glide their private our bodies inside a constrained area, a way to impart the paintings in small regions without reliance on mastering or training in a excellent sort of context. It gives self belief that the Qi Gong art work can be taught in any form of environment.

Practice doesn't have to take area in a hall, dojo, dance studio, or outdoor in a park. Qi Gong can be taught in a broom closet if essential. Teaching in small rooms or restrained areas will, as an trainer, will let you educate and adapt in any other case, permitting you to alter to many strategies of coaching in plenty of regions. Experiencing loads of ways to get preserve of guidance continues the students alert and associated, too, so train in open and confined areas.

Chapter 3: Reflection is Key

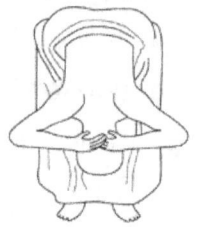

#25: Slow your exercising down.

Slow your workout down. Slow the actions down. Slow the training down. It's higher to deliver the artwork and the teachings of Qi Gong at a mild tempo. This permits time for contemplation, for being within the 2nd, for feeling the strength of the exercise. Slowing down permits the body to re-sample, to tackle board and consist of the moves every from a critical anxious device issue of view similarly to from a muscle reminiscence, structural and connectivity element of view. Slowing down is your body and thoughts and breath coming collectively to permit an issue of exercise session.

Slowing down takes the adrenaline out of the interest and brings you into the center of the movement. It lets in you, as a instructor, to expect, plan, and adapt your teachings without difficulty. You furthermore reap an entire lot of statistics approximately the right forms of moves and postures for your teachings. Slowing down permits you to come to be more aware of the weaknesses and strengths inside a Qi Gong movement.

#26: Practice along with your eyes closed.

Practicing at the side of your eyes closed changes your inner popularity of a movement. It draws your interest inwards. Many instances you can flip what started out as a Qi Gong motion proper right into a Nei Gong movement because of the fact you are aware of and alert in your frame's internal dynamics. I regularly invite my college students to move internal, to close their eyes at the same time as in a standing posture, to try (glaringly in a stable way) moves, paperwork and flowing Qi Gong bodily games. Closing the eyes eliminates visible distractions and brings the frame right right into a extra receptive state. It moreover helps the student to become greater aware of their frame inside the time and space regarding that motion, with out reliance on visual cues.

Closing the eyes gives each other street for inner exploration of the paintings, that's why I regularly schooling posture and movement with my university students first with eyes open then with eyes closed to permit their minds, our our bodies and Qi to build up information approximately in which they'll be inside their very private exercising. This workout is rather beneficial for each pupil and practitioner alike.

#27: Mime your actions.

As a trainer, in case you're in a scenario in which you experience you want to rehearse the moves cleanly and efficaciously, try whenever possible to mime them. Rehearse the ones moves like a dance, without intention, with none Qi Gong thoughts-set, without any deep-seated Qi Gong postures. Mime it like you're rehearsing a hint school dance; this can carry inside the play aspect of the unconscious and could permit you to use a form or a set of sequenced movements. Whether it's far Tai Chi, Qi Gong or another inner martial artwork, this permits you to comprise a fun element.

For instance, I will every now and then workout the dragon form. This is a 5 detail balancing form. It includes numerous special movements, and is used at the side of the five elements from Chinese treatment. It is an attempt to harmonise and stability all the organs of the frame. Sometimes earlier than I practice I will mime all of the actions, then I am aware about collection and float. I make the mime quite and playful. It obtained't always be a high-quality shape, but it lets in get right of access to to the enlargement and space internal my thoughts. It creates an interest of the path and go along with the float from beginning to cease in the key moves, without becoming too concerned in it.

I invite you to apply this on a everyday basis, with whatever, even together together with your martial arts paperwork. Just play with it — it brings in a completely open, unfastened-flowing, revolutionary, and non-restrictive way of remembering your moves.

#28: Repeat perfection.

When you be aware your students start to bypass flawlessly, whilst you spot everything coming together well and sweetly and that they're moving correctly inside the waft, hold those students repeating the movement time and again and all another time, letting them confide in that state of perfection. Because the more they carry out that movement flawlessly, the extra that motion or that posture becomes the default putting in their mind, of their muscle memory, within the cells in their body. It will become the same vintage from which to set all their Qi Gong actions.

It's definitely essential as a teacher to be aware about and alert to perfection and to inspire the repetitive nature of that perfection.

#29: Allow for strength naps.

If you're training frequently or in case you're strolling a retreat, and mainly if you're doing more than a 3 or four day retreat together together with your college students, ensure that you permit for power naps. Do this whether or not or now not or now not it's miles Qi Gong, Nei Gong, meditation or inner martial arts which you are working in the direction of. The purpose for this isn't laziness, it's due to the fact energy naps have been validated to boom the getting to know capability of the thoughts. For instance, for many years in

China, right up till the Nineties in reality, youngsters in pre-faculty and junior faculty were allowed a time after their lunch to nap. This become not simplest for the advantage of their digestion, but additionally to allow them to way what they'd determined that morning and to allow the unconscious thoughts to save it. Part of the cause for sleep is to heal the cells of the frame, allow the coronary coronary heart to slow down and relaxation, and to allow the opportunity organs to detoxify and dispose of waste.

Power naps are a shorter model of a entire sleep, designed at some point of the mind, the mind function, and the processing of the subconscious. This takes on lots of studying in a metaphorical way. The moves, the breaths and postures, may be appeared as an outside manifestation of the talk that is vital for the inner changes to stand up.

So in short, sleep often and energy nap whilst you're schooling tough.

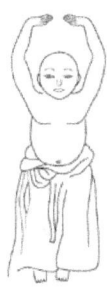

#30: Big it up in studying.

As a instructor, don't be anxious to big it up, to observe huge. That way placed your self in positions in which you're studying with the wonderful, wherein you're in conditions which may be outdoor your ordinary comfort region. Select a teacher who is famend for pushing, encouraging, enhancing and making your Qi Gong huge and further sustainable. That teacher will push you on your restrict. I might probably suggest which you 'huge it up' on a normal foundation. I'm no longer speakme every week, but in reality indoors brief periods of time. Every few years you need to area yourself in the position wherein you're being confronted with a much huge and a much extra centered technique to the work. The effect can be profound and durable.

#31: Reach certainly toward goals.

If you're setting desires collectively together along with your university students, acquire really towards those dreams. All the moves, postures, and go with the flow that you're been offering to them will continuously have a outstanding language method, so as you be conscious your university university students coming near a reason, encourage them with high exceptional vibes. Let them recognise that they may be getting close to their intention. They're no longer going to realize until you tell them, so allow the first-rate remarks go with the flow.

If they're not enticing in the desires you've set, don't make that a lousy deal; allow them to save you, take stock and revisit the movement and postures from every one-of-a-kind difficulty. Or cast off them completely from the art work and get them to do a actually one in every of a type exercising, take their minds some distance from the purpose. When you experience they're relaxed and flowing, return them to the unique purpose. Some university college students reply better to constant stress within the route of a motive whilst others pick out the foot to be on and stale the fuel. It's just like the distinction amongst prolonged distance running and c program languageperiod training. Just make certain to normally attain within the course of the purpose with a high pleasant attitude.

#32: Teach precept without a ebook.

It's vitally vital that as a position version for the paintings, you're able to optimistically explicit the precept of Qi Gong, Nei Gong and inner cultivation with out the usage of a book or notes. When becoming a trainer, you want to examine your idea. You need to find out a way of handing over that idea to the students on your very own phrases. This will imprint for your frame – to your private mind, to your very personal Qi go with the flow – the essence of the art work as it is for you, as it stands on this place, on this time. I'm not saying you have to in no way use written substances or reference books, just which you need to apply your very very personal phrases.

When imparting the concept, try not to break the go with the go with the flow of that transmission. All the super Qi Gong masters, Nei Gong masters and Dao Yin masters transmitted without delay from the coronary heart. The idea modified into so profound and so rooted internal that they spoke freely, without reference, now not first-class inside the elegance, however moreover over a banquet. So even as in any respect feasible, educate precept with out the use of a ebook.

#33: Sandwich the actions together.

If you're coaching a movement fashion of Qi Gong or Nei Gong, try and take a series of actions and layer them. So if there's a center teaching which you want to deliver – as an instance, in case you want to supply a free-flowing, respiratory, on foot fashion of Qi Gong – layer it on top of some status postures or a few clearing Qi Gong. Make high quality which you're constantly alternating between the middle essence of the training and movements in an effort to can help you supply the students decrease lower lower back into their frame or to ground them.

A traditional manner of sandwiching the moves might be first of all a totally grounding posture, which consist of an earth style posture, and then have a look at that with a totally watery movement. Bring it once more to another grounded earthy posture, observed with the useful resource of the use of repeating the flowing water motion, after which perhaps sandwich a few type of clearing to purge any terrible power, and are to be had once more to the recognition another time. The movements are being sandwiched together so the complete turns into a tasty meal for the scholars to revel in in terms of the Qi go with the flow.

Each time they finish their layers, they'll experience coming again to the middle teachings.

#34: Teach the pass 3 instances.

When schooling movement Qi Gong, usually teach the circulate at least 3 instances. Three is a totally vital quantity in Qi Gong. It indicates the philosophies of heaven, man and earth, heaven being the celestial power or the yang electricity,. man being that energy in amongst, and the earth being the yin power.

The guy in amongst is processing the 2 energies on a regular basis, so I might allow the pupil to replicate the flow into as a minimum three times, and on occasion whilst you repeat the motion, repeat it from three tremendous angles or three specific factors or with 3 specific intentions.

My trainer used to mention to me, 'The first time you repeat it, the eyes gain it; the second time you repeat it, the centre gets it and the 1/3 time you repeat it, the heart gets it.' Now, I don't in reality recognise if this is right, but I do recognize that if I repeat anything 3 instances or greater it honestly begins to open up my body and I loosen up and grow to be more comfortable inner what it's far I am looking to teach or impart to my university college college students.

#35: Test your college college students in loads of techniques.

You want to be innovative right here. When I'm trying out my students, I occasionally use the following state of affairs: I ask them to demonstrate an gift movement that I taught them many months in advance, then I test them via slowing the movement down, or through way of asking them to carry out the motion on one leg, or with their eyes closed. I moreover take a look at them with the useful resource of manner of placing them in a standing posture for five or six mins longer than they're used to.

Testing your students is a way of preserving them sharp, maintaining them on their feet and letting them apprehend that you're aware of in which they will be of their exercising. It enables them to apprehend that in the event that they're now not being proper to themselves of their very own exercise, it's going to display in elegance. It can be recognized which you're a trainer who isn't afraid to check your university students.

You also can check your university college students on concept; you can ask them to provide an purpose of additives of their understanding of the artwork so it's now not certainly physical attempting out you undertake.

A in truth real take a look at I discover is meditation. A lot of college students while beginning out can simplest meditate for five or ten minutes, then we feature them up to twenty mins or more. This is a actual test of their staying electricity and perseverance. It's a extremely good lesson for them to have a observe.

#36: Keep your training repetitive and attractive.

I want to maintain my coaching repetitive. I will art work on a concept for perhaps 3 or four months, maintaining it quite cyclical simply so the scholars come to be acquainted with and programmed to the artwork. Each time I supply, I interact them via the use of language this is based for the duration of the manner they studies.

For instance, some of my university college students are auditory, so I trade my pitch and my tone. Sometimes I will shout at them, however no longer aggressively.

Sometimes I'll speak low and smooth. For extraordinary college college students I'll get them to visualize the movements and visualise Qi stepping into their bodies, probable visualise the cosmos, or some factor works for them. Another way of engaging them is via being fingers on, via going round and adjusting and keeping them targeted on me at the same time as supplying the specific discipline that desires to be transmitted. I'm honestly not scared of being repetitive.

You is probably amazed at how prolonged it takes for some college college students to simply integrate frame, mind and spirit.

Chapter 4: Tangible Work

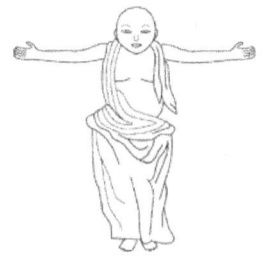

#37: Give purpose for your university students.

They are there for a purpose: to have a examine Qi Gong and find out what they're analyzing it for. For instance, I even have some college university college students who have very low electricity ranges and lead very busy existence. They have advised me that Qi Gong has changed their lives, increased their energy stages and enabled them to live complete lives without being exhausted. I task them by using way of saying, 'Well, possibly you're here to examine this so that you can impart your knowledge and your understanding of the art work, and skip it immediately to those who are in the same characteristic as your self. You're proper right here to investigate and bypass on your getting to know.'

Some students decide they want to become instructors themselves and in that case, I guide them within the direction of that purpose. I inspire them to interact with that cause by using manner of saying to them, 'You've come right proper here for self-development, to beautify your health and nicely-being; now you've placed that you would like to start sharing this work, so I would really like to show you within the path of that intention with the aid of coaching you the art work straight away.' Give them some difficulty tangible. Each scholar has their very personal schedule, have interaction them in that, purposefully.

A lot of my university college students are concerned in athletics. They've come to me trying to beautify their performance. Qi Gong does that for them. Show examples of that on your students. Allow them to sense the art work, change, lighten up, strengthen, improve oxygen waft, de-stress the body, stabilise the knees and the pelvis, and so forth. Give university college students a purpose, then they may dedicate more completely to the work.

#38: Give strong remarks.

It is noticeably important which you are not wishy-washy, announcing matters together with, 'Oh, that end up OK,' or, 'That become better than it changed into 3 weeks inside the past.' That doesn't imply some problem. Give strong remarks. Grab the scholar's interest, name them with the resource of their name, deliver their reputation to what you have got discovered, ask them inside the event that they've discovered it as well, or inside the occasion that they sense any exchange or development. Tell them what you've positioned because of the truth they came within the door, completed their schooling, or within the last 5 mins of doing a particular motion. Being observant and giving comments — whether or not or now not fine or bad — is part of your work as an teacher. Remember, make it tremendous comments. Treat your college students with recognize. They need to be specific at this, they need to beautify, so don't permit them to interrupt out with shoddy exercising. If you revel in it's going to be poor to them, be organization, supply interest to the faults again and again. Be less expensive and respectful, however sturdy.

#39: Always save you earlier than exhaustion.

Never carry your college students to the point of exhaustion. That isn't always the issue of Qi Gong, Nei Gong or inner arts. Even if you are doing a active, hard fashion paintings or movement, by no means bring them to the aspect in which they disintegrate. That defeats the motive of the schooling. You've essentially exhausted them. Not simplest will this demoralise them, it's going to moreover area them in a Qi country in which persevering with to teach is of no further gain to them.

For example, if I'm doing masses of centre-led motion – upwards, downwards, left and proper – or deep postures or centre-losing, centre-developing artwork, and I experience like giving them a workout, I will, but if I begin to see human beings fading off, I prevent. I don't maintain to the factor of exhaustion because of the truth that changes the whole Qi dynamic inside the corporation. It no longer turns into about healing and well-being. Instead, it becomes boot-camp style education. This modifications the way the paintings is introduced and it's going to exchange your dating together at the side of your college university college students. They will begin to see you as someone who isn't always guiding them or most crucial them, but is genuinely there to burn them out. We don't need burnt out university college college students.

#forty: Repeat accurate performances.

After a incredible regular ordinary overall performance of form and posture, ask your university university students to rehearse it via themselves one greater time. You then step away and that they lead the paintings themselves. This lets in them to settle with what they've done, without strain. So, in case you see a scholar execute a shape really properly underneath supervision, supply them a few sturdy fantastic comments and then permit them to rehearse that movement in their very very own time.

This coaching fashion lets in the pupil to take in the paintings, lets in them to settle with the overall overall overall performance, to be assured of what they've completed and to revel in a revel in of fulfillment. Again, it's each other frame-mind-spirit-muscle reminiscence-structural integration style of shipping. By rehearsing the motion themselves, it permits them time for self-statement and to sense snug with their practice, so make certain that a extraordinary general overall performance is usually observed by using the use of the scholar rehearsing through themselves.

#41: End each schooling session on a wonderful examine.

It's essential when you are training to make sure your college students depart the magnificence in a excessive tremendous frame of thoughts. You can also have taken them to the edge and once more, they may be worn-out, some emotions may additionally have come to the fore, troubles may additionally furthermore have rise up, they'll be bodily or mentally stretched, and now you want to make certain that they are leaving your schooling venue with a excellent attitude.

So how can we accomplish this? Emphasise the development and large adjustments in fluidity, motion or stance that you have found inside the session. Again, that is a part of that complete concept of providing strong feedback. Ending on a powerful phrase will help to decorate, the students' notion in their education. For example: currently I became education a scholar who had suffered a couple of injuries to her backbone after being in excessive automobile accidents in the space of 7 years. This female had long long gone via a few Chinese treatment remedy with me, predominantly Tuina and Acupuncture, but turn out to be the usage of Qi Gong as a shape of rehabilitation for her injuries. During this time there has been pain and ache, but moreover moments whilst she felt the ache decreasing or maybe moments when she was clearly pain-loose. So, like any technique, it have become now not smooth, it changed into up and down. It is the equal in all schooling; there is improvement, but it's no longer continually slow and every now and then it can plateau. It have become the equal for her with the healing. But she continuously left feeling slightly better, or able to circulate greater freely. She constantly noticed development. I can also want to make stronger her lessons with positivity, so she observed the effects. It gave her an notion into wherein the paintings may additionally need to take her if she skilled greater frequently at home. Another instance can be the pupil who involves me with knee court cases. When recognition, they locate that their knees are quite sore and after they end their standing postures they have a look at that the knee ache has long gone or is reduced. This reinforces their notion in exercise and training.

Just as in any fitness schooling, there can be an detail of pain. Sometimes we have to recognize that this is a part of the machine. This pain in no way lasts and in reality in some instances, it truely disappears because the person softens and turns into structurally extra aligned at the same time as the energy, the Qi and the blood are all shifting a wonderful deal greater without problems via the gadget.

One terrific concept is more than eight negatives, so if there's any negativity across the paintings, you pretty thousands need to cancel that out. A conventional manner is to save you a consultation with some kind of clearing and grounding art work. That manner the scholar clears the negativity they may be feeling, whether or not the worries and pressures of the day, or concerns over whether or not or no longer they're going to take into account the moves or the positions I've taught them. All of this is eliminated and cleared out of the manner and they'll be left feeling colourful, like they're being scrubbed clean and polished. It takes all of the strain off them. I can't over-emphasise the energy of positivity in this art work. It has a large effect on intellectual fitness and intellectual recovery.

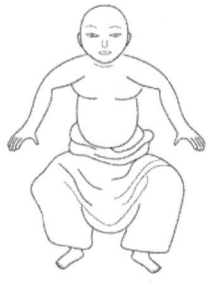

#forty two: Connect with the emotional additives of the paintings.

What can we advocate thru that? Well, that is greater approximately ardour, so when I'm teaching and providing information, I like to go into what I call 'hyper force', in which university university college students can see my ardour rising and might see my enthusiasm for the artwork being projected into my teaching. They can see that I am connecting to what I am doing, and what I am doing is passionately playing my teaching.

Sometimes I tell my college students if the paintings has modified my lifestyles in any effective way, if it has advanced my health, my condition or my intellectual processing. Whatever it's far, I will connect with the passion of that. Being passionate is ready displaying your love for the paintings, displaying how tremendous this form of health safety exercising can be, how it is able to alternate people's lives. Testimonials are also a first-rate detail. Have university university college students supply testimonials in the instructions to suggest how they've stepped forward. This makes them greater obsessed on what they've professional. Get them to attach, if you may, with their feelings.

Ask how they enjoy within the moment; do they revel in focused, do they sense snug? They may additionally feel irritated, they may feel rather frustrated, however don't fear, that's all specific. Connect with that emotion as energy in movement. Be related viscerally, esoterically, and ethereally in the art work. This brings a binding motion, it's similar to the final element that binds the art work together, it keeps it actual – it continues it human.

#40 three: Use brief instructions.

Use brief instructions inside the path of your coaching. That's my philosophy. Over the final thirty-five years of my existence, the pinnacle teachers or instructors I've knowledgeable with have continuously brought guidance in a short, sharp, succinct and right now to the factor manner. This eliminates any confusion and creates readability. It moreover allows the student to hold with their very very personal inner talk. Work out the significance of the transmission to the pupil inside the art work. Vivid and brief instructions are quite difficult to manipulate. It's no longer some thing that typically comes effortlessly. While it's something that requires coaching, we're lucky in Qi Gong as we have a visible element, a bodily problem, and an auditory component within the paintings.

This is why I said in one of the previous tips to bite it down. This tip connects very plenty with chunking down. So if you have, as an example, a complicated arm and frame movement, ruin it down into short, sharp instructions just so the brain can absorb that facts rapidly and make more feel of it. If you over-communicate it, the scholar will become distracted via the amount of language, and it then turns into a lesson in auditory talents in location of the whole integration of physical, highbrow, emotional, and plenty of others.

So with the useful resource of preserving instructions quick, the whole thing may be saved easy, crisp, tidy and to the factor. This also allows location in your college students to ask questions in the occasion that they need in addition explanation.

#44: Use concrete language.

I've had teachers who're very scholarly in their software of the art work and use highbrow, flowery language which fits amazingly properly interior their very own circle. It's like a hidden language human beings with that shape of approach are cushty with. However, whilst you're dealing with a considerable spectrum of the general public, you want to make certain your language is strong, smooth and smooth. It's a piece just like the preceding tip: use quick, colorful, robust instructions.

For example, if you are asking a pupil to face in a certain posture, you need to be clean and urban. For instance, 'We stand on this Wu Ji posture, with our feet parallel, thigh bones straight away below the pelvis, our coccyx is tucked underneath, shoulders are snug, chin is tucked in, backbone is directly, elongated.' It's a listing of easy, honest, concrete instructions. This is ready promoting readability and keeping off confusion. It's additionally approximately building a framework simply so your university college students apprehend you as a teacher and apprehend your style of delivery.

#45: Learn to foster unbiased gaining knowledge of.

This is definitely one among my preferred guidelines. This gadgets you aside on your abilities base, on your education, and in your approach to schooling. I want to take my university students (in particular people who are doing an extended beauty) via a clean warmth up; that is, through a chain of postures and movements to get the electricity up and the blood flowing, and to loosen, melt and open the joints. Then I'll take them to an area wherein I might also teach a shape or a sequence of actions and allow them to pick out a accomplice and teach independently, looking at each one-of-a-kind's actions. I inspire them to art work independently with what they've been given, without the want for my enter.

The benefit of this is that psychologically, it takes pressure off the students. It permits them to discover, with someone of same popularity, the paintings they've been taught. It furthermore lets in them to illustrate in their very own language the work they desire to reveal themselves in. It builds into the muscle memory and the mind the idea that: 'It's OK to take this away and educate with it by myself. I don't need to be reliant on coming to a weekly splendor and most effective education the Qi Gong in that magnificence; I am at a stage in which I can workout on my own.' This establishes the idea that there's a need for impartial mastering in order for development to take area. You will recognize on the day they come to magnificence whether or not or now not they had been education at domestic or not.

#forty six: Learn your paintings deeply.

In distinctive terms, discover it. Explore the artwork, find out excellent elements of the artwork which you had been taught. Don't be afraid to research it. I don't usually imply with the useful resource of searching for quite some books or reading fabric approximately Qi Gong. I suggest thru actually taking what you've been given and trying it in particular strategies. Slow it down, pace it up, breathe in a opposite fashion to what you will typically do, exercise at the side of your eyes closed. Incorporate pretty a few the suggestions I've already given you in this e-book. Mental rehearsal and meditating at the moves you've determined out also are key sports activities. Write down your mind, your thoughts, your feelings, and the feelings that offer you with the effects you need. Re-have a look at the ebook, ask yourself what, if any, issues it has added up for you, what education have been imparted, what feelings have re-surfaced.

Get to recognize what you're teaching, deeply. When you're approximately to impart a few kind of paintings that has been handed right now to you, work with it yourself first, over and over, in lots of unique strategies, in lots of awesome activities. Don't be afraid to paintings with it first in advance than you impart it, because going for walks with it permits it to emerge as ingrained while you train it. It appears greater herbal and related. The diploma of truth you achieve will transmit the ardour, the inducement and the readability you have to your schooling.

#47: Be tough.

Don't be afraid to be tough for your college students. You are there to be a trainer, to be their Qi Gong master, to be their trainer. On occasion, you need to show that you may be difficult, that you may push them. Otherwise, they will in no way pass past twenty or thirty in keeping with cent in their capability. Being difficult doesn't generally imply on foot spherical beating them with a stick or making them do an infinite variety of push-u.S.A.If they get it wrong, it in reality technique being without compromise.

If you're going to make your university college students stand for fifteen mins in a single posture, then lead them to face. Keep them on thing. Determine to take them to that location sometimes and comply with through. It's notable for them, it's a way for them to construct appreciate for you, for themselves and for the paintings. Toughness isn't cruelty; it's far assertiveness, self warranty, and an absolute reality which you've brought your college students to in which you need them to be at that component in time, and that you've imparted precisely what it's miles you need to impart to them forcefully, with self assurance.

#48: Learn it for 8 weeks.

If you have a latest ability, new shape, or new technique of running, studies it for eight weeks. If you're training it, educate it for at the least 8 weeks. Impart that new talent or recovery exercise for your college university college students or have a observe it your self for a duration of 8 weeks. They say it takes thirty days for some element to end up a addiction, so have a examine it till it's miles and then training until you've reached perfection. If you do it for sixty days or extra, you could guarantee it has not quality end up a dependancy, but a way of existence.

Why do I say eight weeks? Eight is the picture of infinity, it's far limitless circles. I assure that if you train this skills for your students on a each day foundation for 8 weeks, it becomes part of their recurring for the relaxation in their lives. It can be very difficult for them to miss it. They may also moreover stumble in a few places on occasion, however usually it will become some thing that is so ingrained that it's natural to them. They don't want to reflect onconsideration on working towards, they surely do it.

#40 9: Don't get caught with some element.

Don't get stuck with one wa of doing subjects. There is a shape known as the Ba Dua Jin — the Eight Pieces of Silk Brocade. It's well-known in Qi Gong practice and it's very famous. It's practiced in masses of precise tactics. Many people teach this shape, and frequently they've continuously finished it the same way; however, if they best ever do it one manner, then that will become the best manner they understand the manner to do it. It can be the most effective approach they ever educate. That sort of paintings can, through the years, emerge as a bit stale.

I continuously encourage my students to try wonderful strategies of doing matters, as an example, a few more breath paintings or a few extra devices of moves, or converting some of the hand positions. Don't get too stuck in the paintings. As we recognise from the I Ching – the Book of Changes – change is the best detail this is regular. I invite you, as the seasons trade, to trade the way you impart your teachings, to stability your college students with the seasons, in case you want. Change your art work as you exchange physical; as you age or as you become bodily stronger or extra bendy, your artwork will alternate and waft.

Never allow your coaching to come to be stale by means of doing the equal element within the identical way, because of the truth you'll emerge as caught. Your Qi will stagnate and your frame becomes rooted in a single detail. Obviously we need a few type of repetition to advantage the perfection I in truth have mentioned previously, but I use repetition with severa exponents. Students attending poorly taught education emerge as set of their strategies. They get snug with a few factor and they're not organized to mix it up, trade it, attempt exceptional methods, or make it extra flexible. Try Qi Gong, Tai Chi with distinctive weapons in place of the same vintage sword. It's important for the person to conform inside the work they'll be doing in order for them to alternate. The very truth that change is normal and power is continuously flowing and reworking makes existence and analyzing greater exciting and exciting.

#50: Love training the fundamentals.

This is some one of a kind appreciably important tip. I located pretty some emphasis on this one. We cited exchange being steady: there are continuously going to be new university college students, new practitioners, and new folks that want to soak up the work. Part of the paintings as a teacher is to embody the basics. The fundamentals are the foundation as a way to supply you in advance as an instructor.

The fundamentals are your protection net even as topics get a piece bit tough or even as you're seeking to impart a few thing that's a chunk sudden.

The fundamentals will continuously be a few issue to deliver your college university students once more to, because of the fact they floor each you and your college students inside the art work.

When I first practised martial arts, I remember education for possibly fifteen years with one teacher. He have become an exquisite exponent of the work, pretty effective, specifically diligent, and pretty tough. But I always felt that not everything turn out to be being imparted.

I take into account one in all his instructors coming over from the Orient to illustrate. He changed into searching at the scholars around us. He need to peer that so a number of the basics, the basics of what they had been supplying were honestly now not being set up. A lot of humans had been without a doubt going thru the motions. He spent 3 hours making us pass up and down the corridor, actually teaching us the basics. But the exceptional factor have become, that for decades after this three hour torture fest, I must experience my martial arts improving, the electricity of my hips growing and my software program of the techniques becoming greater targeted, extra centered.

It is so vital to certainly fall in love with the basics because of the reality once you need them, your college college college students will love them, and this could deliver them a simply sturdy basis on which you could create the maximum cute vision of Qi and get them to embody the paintings from a sturdy stance and base. If the fundamentals are accurate, it continuously makes the extra fanciful moves much less tough because of the fact the form is there. A remarkable foundation will commonly lead and help to take the strain off the pupil greater naturally at the same time as they'll be being challenged. Good basics are a splendid foundation and right foundations lead for a great residence, a house as a way to hold in competition to any stress. That's what you need.

Chapter 5: Qigong

A conventional Chinese workout for curing, preserving, and restoring fitness is qigong

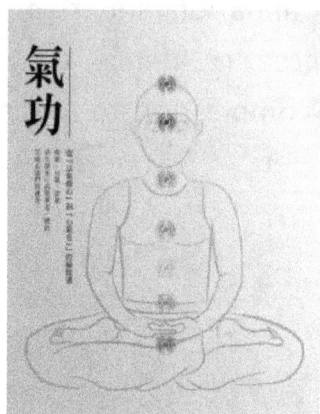

(Qigong). [1] It changed into known as "Dan Dao" in the beyond and refers to a manner for boosting breathing, bodily hobby, and focus (i.E., adjusting the breath, adjusting the body, and adjusting the mind) an extremely good way to strengthen the frame, save you and address illnesses, and preserve fitness. Years of schooling every bodily and mentally to maximize capability

Numerous qigong facts can be determined in medical, Confucian, and Taoist secretaries. In order to carry out the obligations of excavation and sorting, researchers should no longer best have enough records of In addition to having a strong basis in qigong, Chinese medicine, historical Chinese, and modern-day Chinese all require.

The essential difference among qigong exercise and other kinds of exercise is whether or now not the 3 tones are mixed. General sports also have a 3-toned operation content material material, but the three are notable from each different and don't want to be included.

Qigong

A traditional Chinese exercising for curing, maintaining, and restoring fitness is qigong (Qigong). [1] A approach for enhancing breathing, bodily interest, and consciousness (i.E., adjusting the breath, adjusting the frame, and adjusting the thoughts) is known as "Dan Dao" in historic times.

growth physical health, strengthen the frame, and save you and address sicknesses. Years of education every bodily and mentally to maximise potential

Numerous qigong facts may be found in medical, Confucian, and Taoist secretaries. Researchers ought to not handiest have an intensive knowledge of drugs, qigong, historical Chinese, and present day-day Chinese to be able to perform the paintings of excavation and sorting, however moreover they crucial to have a robust foundation in qigong.

The principal distinction among qigong exercise and different forms of workout is whether or not or no longer the 3 tones are blended. General sports sports actually have a 3-toned operation content fabric cloth, but the 3 are first-rate from each different and don't want to be included.

1 Word definitions

Qigong Basic justification for Qigong (3)

According to literature studies, a Taoist monk named Xu Xun wrote the e-book "Jingming Religion Records" within the Jin Dynasty, wherein qigong [qgong] first made an look. Qigong is a thoughts-frame exercising approach that blends the 3 adjustments of frame adjustment, breath adjustment, and thoughts adjustment, in accordance to traditional Chinese remedy.

With the improvement of era, we're now able to draw near qigong the use of the pertinent records of modern generation, so that you can permit us to better recognize the essence of qigong.

Qigong workout is a behavioral remedy that teaches and trains a benign conduct that is right to intellectual and physical health in advance than being subsequently regular through conditioned reflex, constant with the thoughts-set of contemporary behavioral medicine.

The psychophysiological movement of qigong can be defined as: normally the use of autosuggestion as the center manner, to promote cognizance proper into a country of self-hypnosis, and to adjust the stability of thoughts and body through the intellectual-physiological-morphological self-regulation mechanism to attain Self-workout methods for fitness and healing.

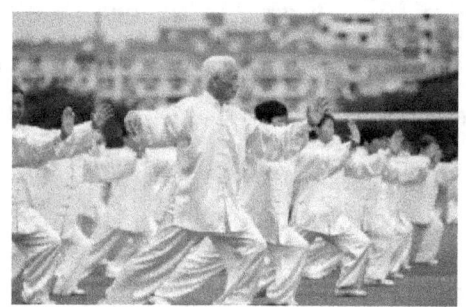

Defining Terms in Taoist Qigong

1. [Nature]: "God," "Yuanshen," which refers to the unconscious, subconsciousness, and innate attention. According to Taoists, the primal spirit is living within the better dantian.

2. "Life," or "Yuanjing," the innate essence; while blended with "Qi" and "Shen," it can

be referred to as absolutely "Essence". According to Taoists, the lower dantian is in which the essence is created and saved.

3. [Pure Cultivation]: The practitioners cultivate through the use of the use of their private "Essence, Qi, and Spirit." It is likewise a natural cultivation in case you exchange "spirit, qi, and spirit" with a person of the alternative sex however do no longer engage in sexual pastime; however, this is called "double cultivation" within the purifying approach.

4. [Double cultivation of life and life]: The practitioner cultivates every his private or concurrent "nature" (spirit) and "lifestyles" (essence).

five. [Double cultivation of the interior and exterior]: The phrases "internal" and "external" talk with the essence, qi, and spirit, respectively, and internal and outside wearing activities are completed simultaneously.

6. [Double cultivation of men and women]: Once each sexes have attained a splendid diploma of inner fortitude, practitioners can exercise "essence, qi, and spirit" through intercourse. Only husbands and other halves are allowed to engage on this form of conduct.

Chapter 6: 2 Development History Qigong

Originating in China is qigong. In China, qigong has a long records. Qigong's number one features in the past have protected

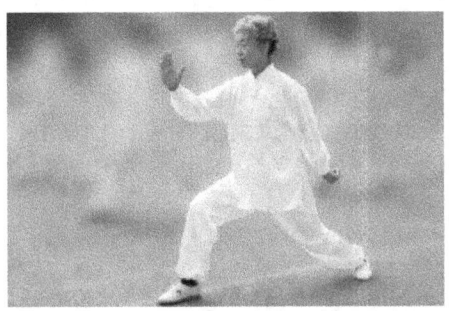

energizing, dispersing, persuading, directing, refining alchemy, cultivating Tao, sitting meditation, and so on. The conventional Chinese medical philosophy of physical care and health is the foundation of the classical Chinese qigong doctrine, which has been round for a completely prolonged period. The "danc" is a part of the unique qigong.

It is implemented as a dance to promote it due to the fact, as it's miles said in "The Spring and Autumn Period of Lu's Family," "the muscle corporations and bones aren't capable of reduce lower back." A part of qigong emerge as encapsulated within the "Daoying Pressing Stilts" at a few level in the Spring and Autumn Period and the Warring States Period. The "Yellow Emperor's Classic of Internal Medicine," a e-book on traditional Chinese treatment, lists cultivation strategies like "lifting the arena, grasping yin and yang, respiratory the essence and qi, independently protecting the spirit, and muscle tissue as one," "gathering the essence and the entire thoughts," "spirit no longer scattered," and others. Lao Tzu makes reference to the breathing techniques of "whispering or

blowing". Additionally, "Zhuangzi" is perception for "bragging approximately breathing, spitting out antique and new, undergo Jing, and hen stretch, handiest for toughness. This person enjoys it who's a guide, body cultivator, and Peng Zu's sturdiness tester. Both the silk e-book "Quegu Shiqi Pian" and the coloured silk artwork "Guoyin Tu" had been discovered in the Mawangdui Han Tomb at Changsha, Hunan Province. The paintings "Chegu Shiqi Pian" drastically speakme introduces the respiratory technique. The "Daoyin Tu" is the primary qigong map. It incorporates forty four images that depict how qigong have become used by ancient human beings

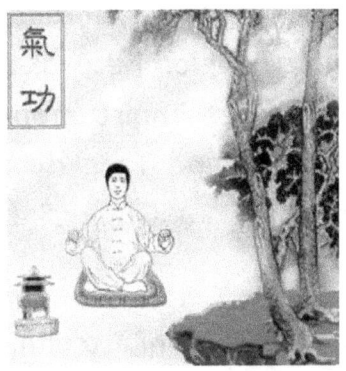

to deal with and prevent sickness.

Development direction of qigong

The later element of qigong is called "dancing," at the equal time as the initial shape has no name. Examples encompass "Abstinence Jue cold and heat, its treatment and appropriateness want to be guided by means of way of manner of stilts" in "Su WenYifa Fangyi Lun" and diverse practices like meditation, sitting and forgetting, fetal breathing, qi movement, convincing qi, regulating Qi, Zhou Tian, Inner Alchemy, and so on. Which are scattered throughout the works of well-known masters from previous dynasties. The time period "qigong" turn out to be at the begin used in the Jin Dynasty e-book "Jingming Religion Records Songsha Ji" through manner of Taoist monk Xu Xun. Following the Sui and Tang dynasties, the "Zhongshan Yugui Fu Qi Jing" facts: "The super

the strategies of qi techniques are comparable, chapters of qigong, but the connotation is not pretty ordinary with what we call qigong. After the Beidaihe Qigong Sanatorium modified into based in the Fifties, it changed into step by step popularized.

People's sluggish summation of severa disciplines, which includes manufacturing, daily life, and sanatorium treatment, consequences in qigong. Physical remedy and qigong treatment are comparable but exquisite from each exceptional. Physical treatment can be a part of it, however it can't take the vicinity of qigong treatment. Always do not forget that qigong makes use of a whole lot of strategies to retrain the mind. Exercises that comprise respiratory assist the coronary heart to acclimatize. The forms of schooling are covered, with inner education serving due to the fact the primary one. Qi in

"Inner qi" and "real qi," that have a deeper connotation, are phrases applied in qigong. At the very least, qigong treatment is a mixture of bodily remedy and psychotherapy, for that reason it has a big form of tendencies.

Jin Dynasty Qigong at its boom degree

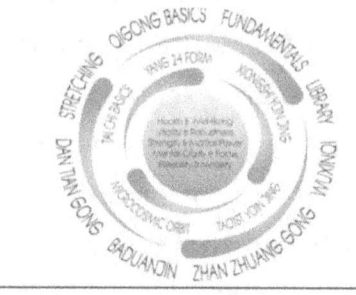

Although Chinese qigong has been practiced for masses of years, the term did now not first seem till an lousy lot later. It first regarded within the Jin Dynasty author Xu Xun's novel "Ling Jianzi." The take a look at decided that this e-book grow to be not authored via Xu Xun as it used severa terminology for qigong that have been never used after the Song Dynasty and therefore could not were written in advance than that factor. Shi Sengyou's "Hongming Ji" regarded within the (Southern and Northern Dynasties) (four collection of Jingming versions),

The qigong is a success with out acknowledging the fortune-telling husband Tao Zhu, in keeping with Hongming Ji, Volume 12.

China's non secular life flourished after the Jin Dynasty. Qigong has been hired by way of religion to demystify it. Qigong's authentic recognition became on growing qi and unique function, which have become very precise and beneficial. However, as quick as it superior into a religion, practitioners pursued cultivation to turn out to be gods, immortals, and Buddhas. The scientific foundation of qigong is lost in this manner. However, in case you have a look at the improvement of Chinese qigong, you will see that severa antique publications with the phrase "qi" of their titles regarded in the Jin, Sui, and Tang eras, on the aspect of

such as "Qi Jue," "Qi Jing," and so forth. The trouble rely number quantity of using and training qi. In "The Classic of Qi," there are a mess of strategies to workout and observe qi. Later religions obliterated qigong, and the phrase itself vanished.

In the Song Dynasty, qigong

According to expert studies, the cultural relic "Warring States Jade Inscription," moreover known as "Xingqi Jade Inscription," "Xingqi Inscription," and "Xingqi Inscription," is an ornament from the give up of the fifth century BC to the start of the 4th century BC this is currently housed within the Tianjin Museum. This is a valuable account of the qigong exercising technique, the earliest and maximum thorough to this point. This hole, impenetrable jade ornament has 45 inscriptions that Mr. Guo Moruo deciphered.

It is stated that The Age of Slavery as follows: "When exercise qi, keep it deep, spread it out, and stretch it down. Fixed topics are solid, solid topics are lovely, lovable subjects are long, extended topics are retreat, and retreat is the sky. The ground gets pounded on the lowest even as the sky is pounded on the pinnacle. You will live to tell the story if you observe along, and you may perish in case you do now not. [4]

Chapter 7: Ming and Qing Dynasties Qigong

During the Cao Wei era, Cao Cao and his son had been both qigong lovers. In order to teach qigong, Cao Cao as quickly as enlisted the help of severa alchemists, which encompass Gan Shi, Huangfu Long, and every exclusive 16 people.

Everyone "breaths and breathes" whilst the owl observes the wolf. Cao himself additionally talked with Huangfu Long about the manner to use Daoyin to boom his lifestyles. It can be the earliest instance of workout deviation in the information of qigong even as Cao Pi, the son of Cao Cao, wrote within the "Ceremony" that "...They had been too impoverished, the air became blocked, and it emerge as Su for a long time." [4]

Current Qigong

Martial arts qigong later superior into qigong treatment, but qigong modified into no longer appreciably recognized. With the blessing and help of the Hebei Provincial Health Department, a senior cadre thru the call of Liu Guizhen prepare a ebook after liberation that summarized his workout and masses of years of clinical experience.

The Ministry of Health's "Qigong Therapy Practice" grow to be officially posted, afterwards translated into different languages, and unfold every locally and internationally. Later, qigong came to be visible as a element of conventional Chinese medicinal drug, foremost to the set up order of qigong sanatoriums and studies facilities that finished massive enhancements in qigong treatment. It is unlucky that the Cultural Revolution sent Qigong, a conventional shape of Chinese way of life, to the bottom level of the 18 levels of hell. Qigong practitioners have transformed into "bulls, ghosts, and snakes."

In a revel in, qigong is "killed" and wiped easy up in this way. The purpose of qigong has seen superb adjustments due to the fact the "Cultural Revolution" ended, and Zhengdao Gong has grown into a first-rate movement.

specific science Everyone has developed a custom. You are conscious that the term "qigong" denotes a unique frame of knowledge. The time period "qigong" is presently used to consult specialized understanding of humans's bodily and intellectual well-being.

The National Health Qigong Management Work Conference modified into hosted in Tianjin through the Health Qigong Management Center of the General Administration of Sports of the People's Republic of China. In addition to representatives from 31 provinces, independent regions, and municipalities across the us of the us, the assembly became additionally attended by means of manner of officials from the General Administration of Sports of the People's

Republic of China, the Sports Bureau of the Xinjiang Production and Construction Corps, and 5 towns which is probably concern to cut up u . S . A . Making plans.

In 2010, Health Qigong showed a pleasant development fashion in some unspecified time in the future of the usa, and large sports persevered all yr prolonged. More than 1 million human beings exercise the counseled bodily video video games, along with Yi Jin Jing, Wu Qin Xi, Liu Zi Jue, and Baduan Jin, at more than 13,000 Health Qigong interest centers throughout the united states of a. The International Health Qigong Federation might be based in 2011, and there were new tendencies in worldwide promoting and exchanges.

roles

Qigong has blessings for treating illnesses in addition to for popular fitness. If the affected person makes a choice to apply qigong as an adjunctive remedy, exclusive qigong need to be decided on for severa situations. Patients with gastropathy and stomach ulcers, as an example, can carry out inner yang qigong;

Patients with most cancers can exercising Guolin New Qigong, Self-Control Qigong, Walking Walking Gong, and certainly one of a type types of qigong; people with excessive blood pressure, neurasthenia, and ache can exercise Relaxation Gong. The advantages of qigong for the aged can also aid patients with neck and shoulder troubles to get better the function of the neck and shoulders. Bedridden patients can choose to intensify the interest to intensify energy.

Qigong is a shape of workout that promotes well being, illness prevention, and sickness treatment thru conscious frame and mind adjustment. To acquire a multiplier effect in next exercising, we need to first comprehend and maintain close to the taboos of qigong health preservation in advance than analyzing the technique itself.

1. Keep "fake" out

In qigong, emphasis is positioned on cultivating "actual qi" and keeping off wrong ideals and movements. Therefore, we need to first discover ways to be a actual character and inform the fact an awesome manner to observe qigong health protection. True qi can best be advanced through a sincere and honest character.

2. Avoid being grasping

Greed is one of the six impurities. Gluttony have to be prevented on the same time as training as it will bring about quite a few troubles and make it now not feasible to reap the exercise state of affairs.

three. Avoid being "moved speedy"

Emotions are the foundation of many physical ailments. The clarification is that human emotions have the capability to intrude with the frame's traditional physiological approaches. When the functions end up disorganized,

There may be sickness. Because of this, qigong practitioners should keep a comfortable mind-set and refrain from being brought on, in any other case the workout is probably vain.

four. Abstain from boasting

In order to avoid obstructing their very own improvement and having negative outcomes, practitioners need to prevent from boasting and depart room for speakme and acting.

5. Prevent "concourse" (different colleges of practice have specific opinions)

To maintain the frame healthy, the essence, qi, and soul of the body are effective. If one does not exercising abstinence in existence, the essence will unavoidably be harmed and inadequate renal qi will result. As a forestall stop end result, it's far advised to exercise qigong to decrease sexual activity. But there are numerous qigong faculties as well.

practices that contradict this (like the Plum Blossom Gate) He made the difference among "jing," a shape of human mind energy, and "sperm." And suitable sexual conduct allows with Gongfa workout.

four Guidelines

Although the thoughts and soul are restricted through their inherent developments and environmental elements, humans can regulate their highbrow and non secular states each consciously or unconsciously. The subconscious and the subconscious are the 2 mental hidden states that aren't aware in human belief. The hyperlink among attention, the unconscious, and the subconscious is the self-order region of the human frame. This dating exists amongst conscious cause, subconscious interest, and unconscious automated movement. Traditional names for the body collection situation consist of "god," "knowledge spirit," and "primary spirit." The

The hyperlink among reputation and the unique spirit is the primordial spirit. The Promise of the God is the physical foundation for instinct, the idea for maintaining consciousness and the crucial spirit, and the memory hint of the beyond existence. In a big sense, the primordial spirit and the primordial spirit additionally can be united and altered by using know-how of the spirit, but in a greater specific experience, the primordial spirit and the primordial spirit can't meddle in inner subjects because of the fact doing so will bring about errors in qigong exercise, fallacious appearance, or misconception.

The holographic lifestyles body that achieves the concord of the three gods and the universe does so via the practice of qigong.

The sublimation and transcendence of existence, this is capable of gift independently and actively for a totally lengthy duration, is what coexistence of lifestyles and existence is. The crucial method for undertaking lifestyles's development is Chinese Taoist inner alchemy. Of course, the four-dimensional statistics our bodies of the solar god and the dead are essentially first-rate, and each are propelled thru antimatter. The internal alchemy workout approach genuinely includes uniting the three spirits with meridian qi, critical qi in desire to rely, and essence qi on the way to aid the soul information that transcends existence.

illustrate

Through unique cultivation strategies, qigong reasons physiological modifications that improve the order and coordination of the frame's tissues and organs' operations. The physiological alterations that emerge from the severa cultivation techniques may even vary. The physiological effect of qigong can be seen in this distinction. Biological strength should have an effect on the frame or devices through intellectual hobby. The psychophysics of qigong.

Qigong gives specific benefits for healthcare. Using the practice of energetic introverted use of aware sports activities, he seeks to reform, ideal, and enhance the existence feature of the human frame and remodel the herbal intuition into the exercise of conscious intelligence. His philosophy is based on the holistic view of existence.

Along with traditional Chinese medicine and martial arts, qigong is regarded as one of the most high-quality components of traditional Chinese way of life and is adored through many people global.

The which means of the term "qigong," which has been used due to the fact antiquity, is doubtful. The phrase qigong turned into not widely utilized in historical times, and the transmission of character physical sports from excellent faculties modified into hundreds greater limited. Modern, at the other. More human beings have heard about qigong than any unique carrying sports. The advertising of qigong with the beneficial aid of Liu Guizhen inside the Fifties marked a turning issue. Liu Guizhen located that traditional physical games are particularly a hit in treating illnesses, as a quit result he

strongly endorsed for the use of conventional physical video games to alleviate ailments. Also known as Qigong remedy. Since then, qigong has evolved right into a way for the general public to recognize the enigmatic universe.

The Liu Guizhen situation is usually a practical one. Additionally, his promotion is quite pragmatic. In the years that located, numerous carrying activities from numerous schools and faculties have been published and orally taught below the call "qigong." but, at the same time as it have turn out to be posted and spread. The majority of those sports activities have had their private ideological components removed. And some noticeably risky material.

Martial arts and qigong each received popularity in the Eighties. Many people are dishonest via improving the qigong's ideological components. Till the Nineties got here to an give up. Following that, both custom and

The qigong stopped. But the popularity of the time period "qigong" has extended. When they promote qigong, Taoism, martial arts, and remedy all mention it.

We can see it in the information and gift of qigong. In this universe, not some thing is possible aside from the secular international. Nothing exists outside of this world. People who came into contact with cultural facts within the beyond knew loads because it come to be no longer considerably allotted. Medicine, martial arts, and Taoism had been all mainly now not like. Cultural information spread hastily after New China modified into installation. It is important to create the broadest generalizations feasible so as for the layman to understand the layman.

about it. It is also natural for experts to change that allows you to adapt to the instances. Experts want to evolve to the times and embrace exchange. Materialism might be this. Things expand in step with their non-public jail tips. Artificially modify the regulation, then restore it to its former form. Also, materialism, this. The worldwide continues to be in huge part materialistic.

We can see it inside the information and gift of qigong. In this universe, no longer whatever is viable other than the secular international. Nothing exists outdoor of this world. People who came into touch with cultural know-how inside the beyond knew a lot because it have emerge as not extensively dispensed. Martial arts, Taoism, and

It emerge as very exceptional in medicine. Cultural know-how spread hastily after New China became installation. Making the broadest possible generalizations approximately the layperson is vital so as for the layman to recognize the layman. It is also herbal for professionals to trade that lets in you to adapt to the times. Experts ought to adapt to the instances and encompass exchange. Materialism could be this. Things broaden consistent with their very personal prison pointers. Artificially adjust the regulations, then restore it to its former form. Also, materialism, this. The global remains in large part materialistic.

Chapter 8: 5 Greeting

The theoretical basis of Chinese qigong is to start with the principles of meridians, acupoints, qi, and blood. Qigong is a excellent jewel within the treasure of Chinese conventional remedy, which incorporates a wealth of data.

residence for Chinese natural medicine. The basis of traditional Chinese remedy and Chinese qigong is the requirements of meridians, acupoints, qi, and blood. Human phenomena like meridians, acupoints, qi, and blood are exceedingly complex. Simply placed, the acupoints function the entrances and exits of the pass of qi and blood, and the meridians feature the pathways for their motion.

The acupoints are gently inspired, and the qi and blood go with the drift without difficulty via the meridians, consistent with the idea of qigong fitness and restoration.

Man, and nature are one.

The holistic vision of the concord among guy and nature, similarly to the harmony among form and spirit, is embodied in Chinese qigong.

1, Chinese qigong places a sturdy emphasis at the harmony amongst guy and nature, their intimate relationship, and the impact of the environment, weather, and other variables at the human frame. The dynamic adaptability among man and nature is as an alternative valued in Chinese Qigong.

2, The concord among man and society is emphasized in Chinese qigong. People's fitness and sickness are right now tied to their social surroundings. Chinese qigong emphasizes the want for social version on behalf of the character.

3, In Chinese Qigong, the concord of shape and spirit is emphasised. A sort of self-bodily and intellectual area referred to as qigong

four, Chinese-inspired health technique. It can beautify no longer incredible the physical capabilities of the human body's body shape but moreover its mental characteristic. The bodily and intellectual talents of the human body are each more splendid via qigong, and the two are interconnected and constrict every other.

Ancient fashion

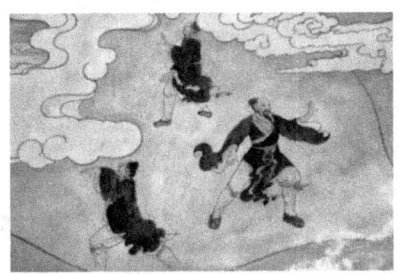

The Han humans have traditionally embraced qigong, which has spawned severa schools of martial arts, Confucianism, Taoism, and medication. Taoist Qigong focuses on the dual development of life and existence, even as scientific Qigong emphasizes health care and extending existence.

6 Tips for Improving Pay hobby on your respiration

convenient and snug

Await results.

comply with the go with the float

in reality

pay hobby

Qigong's biochemical strain

7 classifications

Considering what the sports sports blanketed

It may be separated into active and passive office work. The term "active qigong" describes the self-practice for health and fitness. Passive qigong is a form of remedy that modifies someone's sensible circumstance to address ailments with the help of others. Another call for passive qigong is "outdoor qi" treatment. [4]

from the posture-associated training

It is subdivided into highbrow, bodily, and intellectual modifications. [4]

from the static and physical angles

Static power and dynamic strength are subcategories that may be outstanding.

According to the posture, Jing gong also may be labeled as horizontal, sitting, and small.

There are some kung fu bodily games that may be accomplished at the equal time as sitting, but the majority of kung fu is executed inside the internet style and while shifting.

From the perspective of maintaining the Qi in the frame,

It can be separated into many classes which incorporates Buddhist qigong, Confucian qigong, Taoist qigong, and so forth.

based on how exercise influences the human body

Daoyin Gong Health Gong rubdown

eight Fundamentals

Action posture modifying (Tune-up) A precondition for easy Qigong respiration and the induction of highbrow calm is a glaringly comfortable posture. Physiological components of numerous postures and the posture itself variety.

moreover serves a healing motive. The following postures are often used: reputation, walking, supine, unfastened pass-knee, unmarried skip-knee, and so on.

entering a country of calm (adjusting the mind) A sturdy and quiet united states of america of the united states, free of stray thoughts, is known as coming into tranquility.

It consists of specializing in one element— maintaining the Dantean or paying attention to the breath—weakening the feel of out of doors stimuli, and achieving the united states of being conscious but no longer aware—statistics however not understanding. The cerebral cortex shifts proper into a shielding inhibitory situation. There are 5 widespread strategies to meditation:

1. Be organized to uphold the regulation.

2. Using the hobby method.

three. Use of hobby numbers.

four. Quiet contemplation.

5. Listening technique.

You can start through training the thoughts-abiding approach and then gradually cross without delay to the breathing method or the listening technique, or you could exercise one method constantly. This will rely upon your private opportunities.

Breathing (breathing) Qigong remedy consists of respiratory carefully. Use exercise to head from chest breathing to belly respiration, shallow respiratory to deep respiratory, and in the end practice dantian inhaling your private. There are 8 everyday respiration strategies:

regular respiratory

Refuse to respire.

breathe outward.

Hold your breath.

every mouth and nose breathing.

respiration method referred to as Qi Tong Ren Du Meridian.

underwater breathing

Real Breath

Under the path of the vital principles of kindness and nature, respiration carrying sports have to be increasingly more deep, extended, first-rate, even, and gradual; they ought to no longer be moved quick.

Chapter 9: Action

The maximum crucial shape of kung fu for meditation is sitting pass-legged. The fine of the legs at the same time as sitting waft-legged strongly impacts how masses meditation is practiced, that's critical for a starting. Many beginners are unaware of this, which makes it very difficult to exercising meditation. To improve one's meditation method

nine Editing packages for therapy

Although it's miles supplied, psychotherapy isn't always just like this. In desired, psychotherapy consists of that clinical professional's purpose with sufferers and recommend remedies using language, facial expressions, posture, mind-set, and so on.

Patients in a aware country may be encouraged remedy; sufferers in a hypnotic nation may be recommended remedy through the use of particular induction strategies that generate a hypnotic united states of america substantially like sleep. As a quit cease result, the victim is in no way energetic. Giving complete play to the affected character's subjective initiative is a trademark of qigong remedy.

The affected person can increase strength of mind thru self-exercise and note blessings with the help of the scientific clinical medical doctor.

Connection to Chinese Medicine

The exercise of qigong is crucial to standard Chinese medication.

The techniques, philosophies, and healing effects of the oldest surviving scientific conventional "Huangdi Neijing," which emerge as written greater than 2,000 years within the past, are defined.

All qigong moves were recorded. More than ten of the 80-one chapters of "Su Wen" talk the issue of qigong each right now or not immediately.

It is plain that qigong has advanced proper into a massive scientific treatment method earlier than the Spring and Autumn Period and the Warring States Period.

Chinese medical clinical doctors have given qigong a immoderate priority at some point of the development of conventional Chinese treatment in all dynasties.

Many well-known medical doctors not most effective communicate qigong of their books but furthermore workout it themselves. For instance, in his famous paintings "The Synopsis of the Golden Chamber," famend Han Dynasty medical doctor Zhang Zhongjing wrote: "Only the

Apply moxibustion and acupuncture at the 4 limbs which have heavy stagnation and keep away from growing the 9 orifices.

Here, a form of qigong known as "Dao Yin Tu Na" is stated. According to folklore, Hua Tuo, a famous health practitioner inside the Han Dynasty, wrote the well-known "Five Animals Opera," which continues to be loved via qigong devotees these days.

Wang Tao's qigong has been discussed inside the "Secrets of Waitai," "The General Record of Shengji," and the works "Bao Puzi" thru Hong, "Yang Xing Yan Ming Lu" thru Tao Hongjing of the Southern and Northern Dynasties, "The Origin and Symptoms of Diseases" by means of manner of Chao Yuanfang of the Sui Dynasty, "Prescriptions for Emergencies" through Sun Simiao

within the works of the 4 Jin and Yuan Dynasty masters similarly to within the Song Dynasty.

Only individuals who circulate once more to the watch can see the tunnel. This way that the meridian changes inside the human frame may be positioned as a person plays a sure type of static workout. The renowned Qing Dynasty febrile illness specialists Ye Tianshi and Wu Jutong are every talented in qigong. Discussion and exercise. The famous modern medical doctor Zhang Xichun's ebook "Shenxi Lu" additionally consists of a financial disaster on qigong. The prolonged records of health safety in addition demonstrates the significance of qigong in conventional Chinese medication.

Yin and yang, the 5 factors, the zang-fu organs, the meridians and collaterals, essence, qi, and spirit also are hired as hints in the development of gong techniques and qigong bodily video video games. Qigong is primarily based at the mind of traditional Chinese treatment.

And till prolonged, traditional Chinese medicine philosophy has been the principle deliver of purpose within the lower back of ways qigong works. Of path, whilst you consider that the begin of time, qigong workout has now not in reality been used by medical clinical medical doctors; different schools such as Confucianism, Taoism, Buddhism, martial arts, and others have advanced their very personal interpretations of qigong which may be additionally blanketed in qigong idea.

The consequences of qigong exercising furthermore supply traditional Chinese treatment glowing statistics.

For instance, the 8 incredible meridians precept and the existence gate of Dantian concept, each of which can be notably based totally totally on the exercise of qigong, had been thoroughly described via the medical scientists Li Shizhen and Zhang Jingyue of the Ming Dynasty. Of. The awareness on the usage of the thoughts in qigong is an addition to and improvement of the TCM and emotional theories. In order to certainly understand the general concept of "concord of body and spirit" and "team spirit of man and nature" in traditional Chinese remedy, it's far essential to apprehend the mind-body additives of qigong workout. A radical comprehension of the "Essence, Qi, and Spirit" precept and the Zang-Fu organs' psychological relationships. Excavating

Using qigong along facet medicinal drug, qigong acupuncture, qigong rub down, and specific traditional recovery modalities also can increase medical efficacy and purpose the development of latest treatment strategies.

comparable aspect

Physical interest and qigong are varieties of human self-exertion that every beautify health. Qigong is each different specific shape of physical interest, specially dynamic gong. It is bodily identical to gymnastics, with the exception that the moves are slight and leisurely, if the precise goals for the thoughts and respiratory are eliminated. The 3 factors of "adjusting the frame," "adjusting the breath," and "adjusting the thoughts" are also included in physical exercising. Physical exercising, for example, makes a speciality of "tuning the frame," and the adjustment of

Similar to how prolonged-distance runners ought to balance breathing and pace, respiratory is vital for physical pastime. The guarantee of "adjusting the body" to gain an amazing country is provided thru the proper respiration technique.

Exercise locations a excessive cost at the impact that mental u.S. Of the usa has on physical u . S .. Athletes' highbrow stability affects their aggressive average overall performance in almost all sports activities sports, however to numerous ranges. For example, emotional adjustments may have a massive impact on regular overall performance in sports activities sports sports like taking pix and archery.

In traditional sports sports, qigong and wushu cross hand in hand. The combination of martial arts and qigong is called "outside schooling of muscle tissues, bones and pores and skin, indoors education of breath." The

The health and recuperation results that martial arts have whilst paired with Qigong are what most stand out about their development to within the imply time. Traditional qigong strategies like "Wu Qin Xi" and "Ba Duan Jin" are regularly blended with physical interest.

1. Physical exercise, or "physical adjustment," focuses on "body adjustment." The intention of "breath adjustment" is to make sure the mind and muscular tissues get sufficient oxygen inside the direction of lively bodily interest and to continuously

cast off carbon dioxide from the body. Sports competitions can maintain without interruption if the strength that has been used may be provided in time. In super phrases, its purpose is

to actually engage in physical exercising. Additionally, "alignment" is to ensure that the frame plays flawlessly. This isn't always like qigong. The 3 components of qigong are: "adjusting the thoughts," "adjusting the body," and "adjusting the breath." Of the three, "adjusting the mind" takes the lead and is the maximum big.

"Adjusting the frame" simply serves as a vital precondition for the smooth adjustment of the thoughts and breath. The three truly paintings together to progressively bring about qigong's scenario of tranquillity, and below the steerage of popularity, self-adjustment and workout of the frame's inner features are finished.

Through a selected mental procedure, the physiological nation of the frame is altered.

to fulfill the aim of healing ailments and improving the frame.

2. In evaluation to bodily hobby, qigong emphasizes the effect of humans's intellectual states on human fitness and places a robust emphasis on enhancing one's private physiological strategies through proactive self-intellectual sports. The physiological capability of the human frame may be inspired and advanced within the situation of qigong coming into the though united states of the us, and this can assist to enhance the frame and deal with ailments.

3. Breathing is a necessary part of qigong exercise, it really is completed because the practitioner enters a despite the fact that circumstance. In order to keep calm and rest, the whole body should circulate in unison even as breathing lightly and slowly

to lower oxygen consumption, coronary coronary heart charge, and blood stress.

coronary coronary heart price.

Enhance preferred bodily fitness; that is going hand in hand with extremely-modern bodily interest, which speeds up breathing, will boom oxygen consumption, quickens coronary coronary heart rate, and quickens blood pressure, speeding up the metabolism of particular frame additives and inflicting the body to growth flawlessly according with requirements. The difference.

It is a giant capabilities that is extremely good to our u . S . A ..

2. There are eleven fantastic varieties of fitness qigong selling strategies recognized thru the Qigong Center of the General Administration of Sports of the People's Republic of China.

Chapter 10: Balanced respiratory, yin and yang

As we observed in the economic disaster devoted to this, records the idea of Yin-yang can be very essential inside the Luohan gadget.

But now not simplest can we want to understand its content material, however we want to furthermore apprehend its relationship to the human body and its software to the physical games and movements we perform in our exercise.

1.A BASIC EXERCISE

The first exercise we are going to observe is supposed to familiarize ourselves with this idea, a manner to apply it to our exercising and experience its effects on our body.

To start, we're capable of adopt one of the beginning positions. Any of them can be useful. Personally, I like to exercising this exercise within the repute function, however any of the alternative sitting positions can be used. We can pick any of them counting on the sports we are going to art work on after this one, so we do now not want to be changing.

As I typically begin the usage of this exercise at the start of the elegance or training consultation, as a part of the high-quality and comfy-up, it's miles extra comfortable for me to do it reputation up, even as you take into account that it's miles going to be located by using others within the same characteristic. If we prefer to do it at the prevent of the consultation, precisely for the alternative, to loosen up and skip lower back to calm, it can be an extremely good idea to do it sitting down.

Let's do it;

BALANCED BREATHING

Since we already truly understand the standards of Yin and Yang, we will define balanced breathing as the only that has a neutral effect on our organism.

With it we do now not intend to spark off (yang) or sedate (yin), what we are searching for is a neutral or balancing impact. We are searching out to sell the motion of power, however in a balanced way.

To reap this, we are capable of focus on making our suggestion last up to our exhalation. And as a reference, we can depend to a few whilst inhaling, and we are capable of moreover keep in mind to 3 on the identical time as breathing out. Obviously, this rely of three may be faster or slower counting on the lung ability of genuinely anybody. It is in truth a depend of counting just so belief and expiration very last the identical time.

Balanced respiration is a number one technique at the way to help us attention, lighten up and understand our body similarly to do away with tensions and sell proper flow of qi.

We have to preserve in mind that we need to in no way pressure our breathing. Normally, it's far simply useful no longer to fill our lungs even as breathing in over 70 percent of their capability. This will keep away from unnecessary anxiety and a higher use of the inspired air.

Try to make an notion filling the totality of your lungs. You will proper now have a look at which you disturbing excessively and are compelled to allow the air out quick, dropping control of the exhalation.

Our cause is to understand the breath and learn how to manage it and "play" with the four ranges that compose it to collect one-of-a-kind responses.

If in choice to filling the lungs truly, we do it approximately 70 percent, we're capable of apprehend that we are capable of preserve the air lots longer if we want after which we are able to manipulate the exhalation a bargain higher and make it longer, shorter, immoderate or tender in line with our will.

Practice

Adopt one of the two beginning positions we've got got visible. As I simply have described in advance than, you could stand, or sit, whichever is more cushty for you.

Allow yourself some seconds, or as plenty time as you remember critical, to focus on your position, reading the factors we observed; toes shoulder width aside, decrease again right away, hands snug, and gaze immediately beforehand. You can hold your eyes open, but I recommend you to close them slightly, it will assist you isolate yourself from the out of doors and recognition on your self.

Once you have got got got regulated your body, we interest on your respiratory. Breathe in thru your nostril and breathe out through your nose or mouth, whichever is extra snug for you. Feel your breathing and be privy to its four levels that observe every other in a cyclical manner (1.-breathing in, 2.-pause, three.-respiration out, four.-pause). Gradually make your respiration deeper, longer, smoother and extra rhythmic, warding off overfilling your lungs and controlling that even as you breathe out, no longer all of the air comes out right away.

Do now not worry if earlier than the whole thing you get distracted or your mind take you a few other vicinity. When you recognize this, absolutely interest again in your respiratory.

After some time, which may be numerous mins or via in truth working towards a few breaths, we becomes aware of the period of our respiration.

Let's attempt to make the inhalation and exhalation final the same amount of time.

As a guide, you can rely to 3 on the inhale and additionally to a few on the exhale.

This may have a independent impact on qi. We surely control to make it circulate (in addition to all the benefits that respiration sports sports can carry us), however in a extra independent way.

When breathing in, we're capable of phrase how we obviously stretch the spine and amplify the body, as although we had been growing, despite the fact that occasionally it's miles a very subtle movement and almost no longer vital.

When we exhale, we are able to test, moreover virtually and with out forcing, that the frame has a bent to loosen up and return to its preliminary characteristic. Do now not pressure it, cognizance first nice on respiration, and then you'll be aware how the body by way of manner of using itself makes those actions. If, through the years, you need to intensify this sensation a hint, you can stretch your knees whilst you breathe in and bend them a hint whilst you breathe out. Thus, the complete frame will stretch slightly on the inhalation and loosen up on the exhalation. But as I indicated, all this need to be very diffused and now not forced. It must be a impact of respiratory.

YANG BREATHING

In this form of respiratory, we are able to make the inhalation longer than the exhalation. A similar effect would furthermore be completed with the aid of setting extra emphasis on the inhalation (strengthening it).

To acquire our intention, we would consider to four on the in-breath and three on the out-breath.

The effect we accumulate with this form of respiratory is yang art work; elevating energy, stretching our frame, accelerating circulate, and so forth.

Practice

As with the previous workout, pick out the beginning function that is maximum snug for you. Allow yourself a piece time to focus and regulate your respiration. After some repetitions, interest on the timing and make the inhalation a hint longer than the exhalation. As I showed, a excellent manual may be to rely to four on the inhalation and 3 on the exhalation.

This may additionally have a greater toning effect, extra yang; it's going to assist to prompt us, to growth our strength, to revitalize us, and many others.

YIN BREATHING

With this type of breathing we get the other effect, we are capable of get a yin exercising; decreasing the power, fun the frame, calming the flow into, and so on.

To attain this, we are able to make the inspiration shorter than the exhalation. On this event, it would moreover be useful to location extra emphasis on the exhalation (strengthen it or greater said).

Returning to the mathematics, we are able to rely to 3 whilst breathing in and to four even as respiratory out.

Practice

Exactly like the previous ones, after adopting a beginning posture, regulating and listening to our respiratory, we're capable of popularity on the instances, counting now up to three whilst breathing in and as a lot as four while breathing out.

With this, we get a more enjoyable, calming and sedative effect. A more yin effect.

Only with this type of simple breathing and information the concept of yin and yang, we've were given had been given already seen how we are able to get exquisite results on our frame via way of creating small versions in the length of the notable tiers of breathing.

It is simple, smooth, however exceedingly useful for our workout. What we've got just visible applies to most of the sporting activities, and information it successfully, we will adapt them to our goals, relying on whether or not we are trying to paintings in a more energetic, stimulating, extra exciting, softer manner or truely want to do a more balanced paintings.

On events whilst we want extra power (while we're worn-out, apathetic, and so forth.), running toward yang kind respiration can assist us.

On the alternative hand, in conditions wherein we need to lighten up (because of strain, anxiety, fear, and lots of others.) inhaling a yin way may be beneficial.

If we really need to mobilize energy, attention the mind and gain our general health and well-being, balanced respiratory may be appropriate.

There is another manner to convert our independent respiratory into yang or yin:

Faster respiration will pressure us to do more shallow respiratory, consequently reaching a yang impact, helping to raise our coronary coronary heart charge, our strength, and so forth. On the opposite, a slower respiration will lead us to make a deeper breathing, with which we will advantage a more Yin impact; more rest, decrease our coronary coronary heart fee, and so forth.

1.B - BREATHING EXERCISE USING ARMS

Once we have were given had been given determined to control the breath, to paintings it in a balanced manner, yin or yang, depending on what we want to gain, we're capable of add the motion of the arms.

To do that, we are able to undertake the beginning position status. As continuously, we are able to do a chain of unbiased breaths to loosen up and cognizance on what we're going to paintings on next.

To start with this new exercise, from the beginning function we are able to place the fingers coping with upwards, inside the the

the front of the frame, beneath the navel, with out touching and with the arms snug, as we are capable of see inside the image.

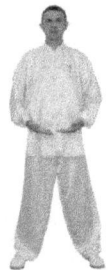

The rest of the frame remains the identical.

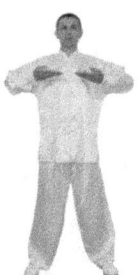

From this role we are able to start to inhale, elevating at the same time the fingers in the the front of the body till they attain approximately the height of the shoulders.

Once we gain this problem, with a pronation of the forearm, we vicinity the palms going

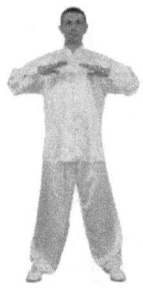

via downwards.

From proper right right here, we exhale lightly at the same time as decreasing our fingers in the front of the body, as despite the fact that we desired to push a few aspect (but without putting pressure).

At the equal time, we will additionally barely bend our knees and sink the coccyx downwards. When we end breathing, the fingers have to be on the quantity of the navel or some centimeters lower. Legs and fingers bent. Back without delay, however snug. Look at once in advance, a bit down as though we were looking at a much off factor at the ground (approximately 15-20 meters

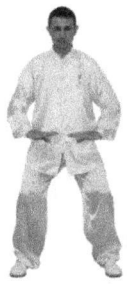

away).

From this component, we cross back to vicinity the arms up with a supination of the forearm. Then we breathe in even as stretching our legs and lower returned.

At the equal time, we enhance our fingers and our gaze, an remarkable manner to preserve ahead however now slightly upward. When we finish breathing in, the hands are at shoulder degree as in advance than and we repeat the whole process.

In this manner, at the equal time as we breathe in, we stretch our legs and returned, enhance our hands and gaze.

During the pause, we turn our palms. On the exhale, we bend our knees, loosen up our backbone and gaze, and decrease our arms. At the pause, we turn our arms.

In this workout we will include a greater artwork of the shen, this is to say, of our thoughts or interest.

When we breathe in, we have to have the feeling of developing, maintaining our toes firmly on the floor. We can direct our hobby to the bai hui element, positioned within the maximum part of the pinnacle, and experience the way it moves upwards and we stretch the spine.

At the same time, we are capable of do not forget that we are maintaining some thing heavy in our arms and we are lifting it up with the electricity of the whole frame (the extension of the legs and the backbone, and with the fingers). All this with out putting anxiety; it's far a bit of creativeness or recognition an great way to help together with the movement and breathing to elevate all the qi (electricity-feature-interest) upwards.

When exhaling our reason is to press down with the hands (I insist, with out anxiety, it is a highbrow paintings), on the identical time we experience how we sink the groin and coccyx, for this reason growing the stress on the soles of the toes.

This workout can be practiced with any of the 3 kinds of respiratory that we have were given seen and worked in the preceding exercise. That is, we are able to artwork it in a balanced way, in a yang or yin manner counting on the impact we need to gain.

As earlier than, if we artwork it in a balanced manner, after breathing in and out, the body may be precisely similar to at the same time as we commenced out.

But if we art work it in a yang way, we can see how every repetition of the exercise the body may be a chunk greater stretched, annoying or energetic. If we art work with yin respiratory, the alternative will display up. Each repetition we are able to be enjoyable and flexing our frame greater. In truth it's far some thing diffused, but if we repeat it numerous instances it begins offevolved to be positioned.

There isn't any defined or appropriate sort of repetitions for every workout. Everything will rely upon the volume and revel in of the practitioner.

As a massive rule, the balanced exercising may be practiced as normally as we want (typically in the diploma of exercise of every one). For the yin and yang versions it would not be handy at the start to replica it greater than 4-five times because of the fact as we've got seen, each repetition the body has a tendency to stretch or loosen up, and any excess may be wrong.

Chapter 11: Work of the three heights in a sitting function

In previous chapters, we've already seen that the Luohan tool seeks to increase and decorate the three treasures of health. We have additionally located that we will do this through movement, breathing and recognition, and that there are various critical elements or factors as a manner to direct or control those three techniques of education. These are the gates (movement), the jiaos (respiration) and the dantian (interest).

We additionally observed that we may additionally want to divide the frame in 3 zones and that every of them had its private gate, jiao and dantian, which want to paintings in a coordinated way for a accurate and effective training.

Once we've decided out to control our herbal or linear breathing, and to workout it in a yin, yang or balanced way, our critical purpose now is to discover ways to train every of the three heights.

In the subsequent exercising, we can learn how to pick out out each of these 3 zones and to use their corresponding critical factors (gate, jiao and dantian) successfully. We will discover ways to bypass, breathe and recognition on the work of every of these heights.

This time, it's miles essential to begin within the sitting characteristic. This will allow us to popularity at the torso, which can be the regions we are going to paintings on. We can do this on a chair or at the floor with our legs crossed. For most humans, sitting in a chair, as described within the corresponding phase, will be an lousy lot less complicated and extra snug.

2.A- To train the better area

To begin, we take a seat down down effectively, as we observed within the chapter on starting positions. This time, the fingers need to rest at the thighs with the fingers dealing with upwards.

As normal, we're able to do a chain of breaths to lighten up and focus at the exercise we're about to do.

Once we've got executed the ones breaths, we reputation on the pinnacle vicinity motion.

Upper Gate;

In the begin characteristic, we are managing beforehand with the lower back without delay. We direct our hobby to the better gate, simply among the atlas and the occipital. Trying to make the movement get up from this component, with out transferring the rest of the cervical, we bypass the top, elevating the chin and stretching the anterior neck muscles (this is precisely what we are searching out) till we look up 45 stages. At the identical time, we're able to be aware how subtly the shoulders are pulled backwards and outwards, barely widening the region of the clavicles and higher sternum. We will call this "beginning the gate", on this occasion,

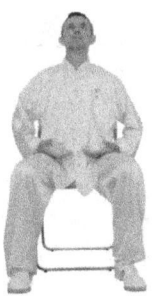

the pinnacle one.

Then, taking the top gate as a reference component, we gently go back to the preliminary position, with our gaze dealing with earlier and our shoulders comfortable. We will call this "ultimate the gate".

We repeat numerous instances, normally 3 to five instances.

We have already determined to apply the top gate, which directs the motion of the

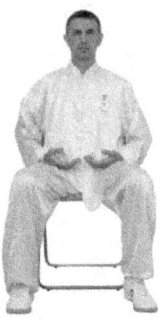

top. In exceptional terms, even as in the Luohan machine we skip the top, we do it from the higher gate.

Upper Jiao;

As we noticed in the theoretical phase, the training of the one-of-a-type jiaos can be completed with the breathing.

What we are going to do next is to learn how to direct the air to the pinnacle Jiao, that is to mention, to the pleasant a part of the lungs. Therefore, it's miles going to be a superficial respiration and, as a surrender give up result, quite brief.

From the beginning function, we perform the motion of the higher gate and, consequently, of the top. At the identical time, we breathe in through the nose, specializing in using pleasant the maximum superficial element. Then, at the same time as we cross again to the preliminary role, we exhale the air thru the mouth, emitting the "U" sound.

The initial motion of the head have to coincide with the inhalation and the pass back movement with the exhalation.

In addition, while breathing in, we are able to press lightly with the tongue the top palate and at the same time as respiratory out we are capable of simply lighten up the tongue returning to its natural role.

Upper Dantian;

As we've got already visible, within the Luohan gong art work, the dantian are the zones to which we are able to direct our hobby to the precise carrying sports.

From the start function, we start the motion of the pinnacle, generally from the gate. At the identical time, we breathe in thru the nostril, seeking to fill the top part of the lungs. And now, at the same time, we direct our hobby, our purpose, to the better dantian. When we come decrease back to the preliminary role, we breathe out through the mouth with the sound "U" and loosen up our thoughts, our cause.

In a way, it' s approximately our motion, our respiration and our cognizance or goal shifting at the same time. Jing, qi and shen must be coordinated. This is the essential element to Luohan and what is going to make its work effective.

Sometimes it's far going to be the movement that directs or "drags" the alternative . At different instances, it will likely be the breath that leads the exercise and at others it'll in all likelihood be the mind or purpose. But whichever one initiates the movement, all three need to be in unison.

Key elements

•The critical goal of the exercise is to learn to direct the respiratory to the extremely good part of the lungs. To engage the most superficial and decrease ability a part of the lungs. When acting the movement from the gate as we have described, we're able to word how the anterior neck muscle groups stretch and slightly beautify the clavicles, permitting or facilitating the air to go to that lung location.

•Therefore, the most important points are the proper use of the gate, and respiratory most effective with the very pleasant a part of the lungs, with out the usage of different regions.

This form of respiration is not the maximum suitable for our fitness and well-being, and we need to no longer exercise it for a excessive form of repetitions, thinking about the reality that it may produce a "hyperventilation" in which a massive elimination of CO_2 occurs inside the exhalation and developing the proportion of oxygen in the blood.

This is clearly an exercising to learn to artwork this region in isolation and to consciously convey the respiration to this pinnacle. Four or five repetitions consistent with schooling session is probably enough.

Common errors to avoid;

•Avoid hyperextension of the cervical backbone. The motion need to be simplest of the better gate and therefore we pleasant beautify the gaze handiest 45 levels. To circulate any higher need to imply an excess of tension.

•It is probably a chunk the equal when descending. At the start of the exercising, the gaze is inside the front and on the surrender of the workout it have to remain the identical. It might be very commonplace to decrease it more, which is wrong. Now we're jogging all the time inside the better place and if we direct our gaze downwards, this motion will visit the lower zones.

•Another commonplace mistake is to make the breath too prolonged. Now we're learning to paintings each peak one after the other and we attempt to direct the air to each honestly one in every of them. This time we are directing the air handiest to the top zone, the maximum superficial location of the lungs and consequently with little air we're capable of fill it. This is a brief breath. If we maintain inhaling, we're capable of most probably fill specific heights and therefore a part of our paintings might also additionally go to those distinct zones.

•Finally, the movement we've had been given defined of the shoulders may be very diffused and it is possibly that earlier than the whole thing we are capable of no longer phrase it. We must not strain it at all. In truth, it's miles a result of the movement of the gate and specially of the air that enters the quality a part of the lungs, which widens that location (consequently the moderate movement of the shoulders) and will increase the collarbones. As I stated, we ought to no longer pressure it and circulate the shoulders intentionally, however in a herbal way due to what modified into described above.

2.B- To teach the Middle place

Once we have completed running the top location, we bypass directly to learn how to use the center quarter, that is, the way to use the gate, the jiao and the middle dantian.

To do that, we maintain in the identical seated function, but this time we rest our fingers on our thighs except that the palms are going through downwards. In truth, what we relaxation on the thighs are the wrists and the arms are touching the internal of the thighs, looking down, however a bit outward. The arms and shoulders continue to be comfortable, the lower again without delay and dealing with in advance.

We now reputation at the middle area.

Middle Gate

We attention on the center gate positioned the various 1/3 and 4th dorsal vertebrae. Taking this aspect as a reference, we begin an extension of the dorsal spine, taking this

171

spot, meaning the gate, slightly in advance, inside the path of the anterior part of the spine. As a impact of this, we can examine how the chest expands. To the edges and to the the the front, widening the rib location and moreover the sternum.

We may also even look at how, even though it's a long way very slightly, how the elbows float to the the front and components. This has to be a result of the movement of the gate and consequently of the chest. We should not strain it and skip the elbows

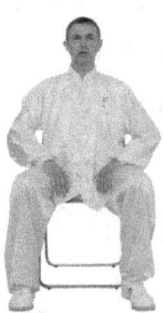

independently.

We will name this motion "beginning the gate", in this event, the center gate.

Then we will cross again the gate to its initial function, consequently exciting the dorsal spine and last the chest, ribs, and sternum region. The elbows can even flow again to their initial function.

This motion is known as closing the center

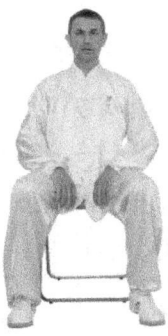

gate.

During the complete exercising, every at the same time as putting in place and very last, your eyes will remain looking right now earlier.

Middle Jiao

We have already learned that to educate the jiaos we do it through respiratory. Therefore what we are going to do is to direct the air to the center area of our lungs. It will not be the internal most, but it is not as superficial as in the pinnacle breathing.

From the begin function, we carry out the gate movement described above. At the same time, we breathe in, however this time via the mouth, with the lips inside the equal position we use whilst making the "Ooo" sound. This, together with the boom of the chest and ribs produced through manner of the movement of the gate, will purpose the air to be directed to the middle location of the lungs. As we defined in the pinnacle sector physical sports activities, the motion of the gate and the inhalation ought to be on the equal time. In this manner, the growth of the entire middle area is an awful lot more effective in bringing the air to that vicinity.

Then, and moreover on the same time that we "near the gate" returning to the initial function, we release the air, moreover through the mouth and with the identical function of the lips. But now, further, we additionally emit the sound "Ooo....".

To artwork on the middle jiao, the tongue remains snug all the time in a natural manner.

Middle Dantian

From the start role, we carry out the motion of "starting the gate" at the same time as respiration as truely described. At the equal time, we placed our "mind", our goal within the center dantian. This, along facet the movement and respiration, will help to direct the qi, the energy, the hobby there.

By remaining the gate and respiratory out, we lighten up our "mind", our attention. In this manner, we assist the qi we've got have been given directed there to circulate in the direction of the region.

Key elements;

Proper use of the middle gate will set off the external intercostal muscle groups, which convey the ribs and sternum, consequently growing the diameter of the rib cage. This boom in quantity creates a horrific strain that reasons air to go into the region. For a majority of these motives, it is crucial to carry out the movement from the gate.

Common mistakes to keep away from;

A not unusual mistake is to transport the fingers independently from the body. The motion want to continuously begin on the gate. This reasons the chest to boom, and this motion eventually finally finally ends up undertaking the palms.

2.C- To educate the lower sector

We have already discovered the way to art work the better and center zones. Let's bypass now to the decrease one.

To do that, we're capable of adopt the same sitting function, but this time we're able to relaxation our hands on our knees with the hands, now, completely down. As normally, again at once, shoulders and palms comfortable and look right away earlier.

We will reputation on the whole decrease place.

Lower Gate

Let' s consciousness our interest at the decrease gate. As we did with the middle, we begin an extension of the lumbar spine from this element, bringing the lower gate barely ahead at the identical time. This will reason the lower stomach to boom within the direction of the the the the front and the knees to split slightly. At the same time, we are able to deliver the chin towards the chest, stretching the cervical area and blocking off the better area. The eyes looking about 45 tiers downward. We will name this movement "establishing the decrease gate".

Subsequently, we are able to relax with the useful useful resource of returning to the preliminary characteristic, thrilling the lumbar backbone, bringing the knees nearer collectively and turning our gaze to the the the front. We will name this "final the decrease gate".

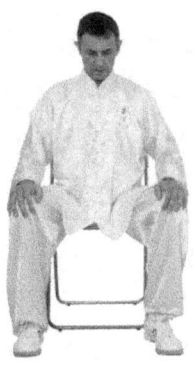

Lower Jiao

To paintings the lower jiao, we're capable of direct the air we inhale to the decrease quarter.

From the begin function, we carry out the decrease gate movement as we've got were given found out. At the same time, we do an concept, additionally via the mouth, but this time the location of the mouth is much like the only we use at the same time as we make the "A" sound.

During the foundation we region the tongue at the decrease palate, urgent with the end of the tongue the inner a part of the lower the the front enamel.

Subsequently, and coinciding with the motion of closing the gate, we release the air, moreover through the mouth, adopting the same function that we use even as we emit the sound "Aaaee". That is to say, a completely open "A" that at the give up appears to combine with the "E".

During exhalation, the tongue remains within the identical position as while we breathe in.

Lower Dantian

From the initial function we flow into the decrease gate at the identical time as breathing in for that region. Now, at the identical time that we do all the above we positioned our shen, this is, our thoughts or goal in the lower dantian, for this reason assisting the qi to visit that place.

When we near the gate and release the air, we lighten up our attention assisting the qi that we have got taken to the decrease dantian to circulate at a few degree in the decrease place.

Key points;

This is the inner most respiratory and the one that might be the maximum tough to acquire. Using the diaphragm efficiently is essential and for this, as general, the right use of the gate will help us. It is essential to tilt the chin down (up to forty five tiers), as this can block the pinnacle vicinity and assist the air to visit deeper elements. It is likewise useful to put our hobby on the decrease dantian.

When doing the gate motion we noticed that as a stop result we growth the decrease stomach and slightly separate the knees. The hands are nonetheless resting on them and therefore also are separated, but the elbows live cushty and ought to no longer be opened, to prevent the air from going to the center vicinity.

Common mistakes to keep away from;

A commonplace mistake is to magnify the motion of the chin. With this motion, we need to assist the air visit the lower area and on the equal time focus on that component. But if we lower it over 45 ranges or pressure this movement an excessive amount of, we are able to put a similarly of hysteria within the pinnacle place (cervical and neck) in an effort to purpose the qi to move incorrectly to that place, in addition to complicate the breathing.

General issues

In this workout, we discover ways to discover and use each of the 3 heights. For this, we use the gate, the jiao and the dantian similar to each one of them. They will assist us manage and direct the movement, breathing and attention to artwork on every area.

It is essential to understand that the three factors want to be finished on the equal time. In the Luohan tool it's miles fundamental that the 3 treasures, jing, qi and shen pass in coordination. They have to no longer be separated or pass their separate techniques.

And that is what we should gather with this series of physical sports. We must open the gate, breathe in, and cognizance at the dantian at the equal time. Then, moreover on the identical time, we can close the gate, breathe out and lighten up the mind. That is what's going to make our exercise of Luohan as a qigong device effective.

Later we will see how inside the fashion there are wearing events in which one of the 3 factors or treasures directs the opportunity . There may be physical video games in which the movement initiates the movement and the breath and thoughts look at. At exceptional instances, it will likely be the breath that leads the movement and at others it'll probably be the thoughts that directs the opportunity treasures.

This will assist us emphasize the paintings of each of the three factors, and consequently certainly one of them takes on more prominence and directs the alternative . But within the same manner, the three ought to be coordinated and at the same time. Although one is the number one one and the only who initiates the movement, the opportunity two have to study him and work at the equal time. The truth that there can be one main the exercising does not suggest that the alternative must not art work on the same time. In reality, it's miles some aspect very diffused that we are capable of see in greater superior practices.

For the instant, what we intend with the ones first physical sports is to learn how to teach the three treasures and the 3 components that represent them at the equal time.

www.ingramcontent.com/pod-product-compliance
Lightning Source LLC
Chambersburg PA
CBHW071339120626
46546CB00002B/619